D1740573

Hair Psychology
My Glory, My Hair, My Loss

Written By Fay Michelle
Created With Support From
Comfort Legacies
Jacqueline Nero-Douglas
www.comfortlegcies.com
comfortlegacies@gmail.com

Hair Psychology-My Glory, My Hair, My Loss

Written by Fay Michelle

Written by Fay Michelle
Created With Support From
Comfort Legacies
Jacqueline Nero-Douglas

Hair by it's definition is an appendage of the skin. Boy, do we love this appendage! Losing hair can break us down. During hair loss times, we can experience decreased confidence, anxiety and depression.

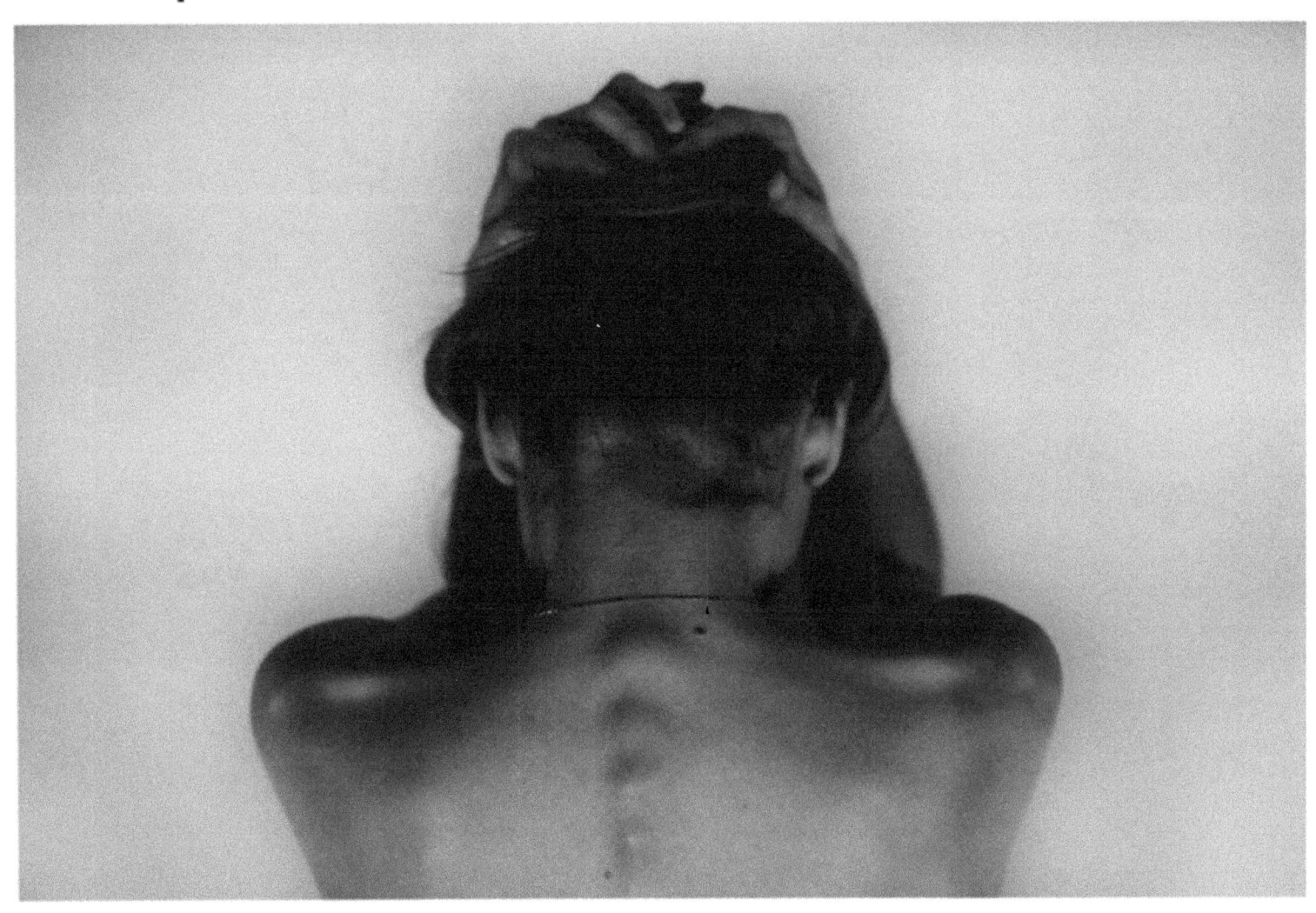

Losing hair can cause excessive worry. Stress and hair loss are related.

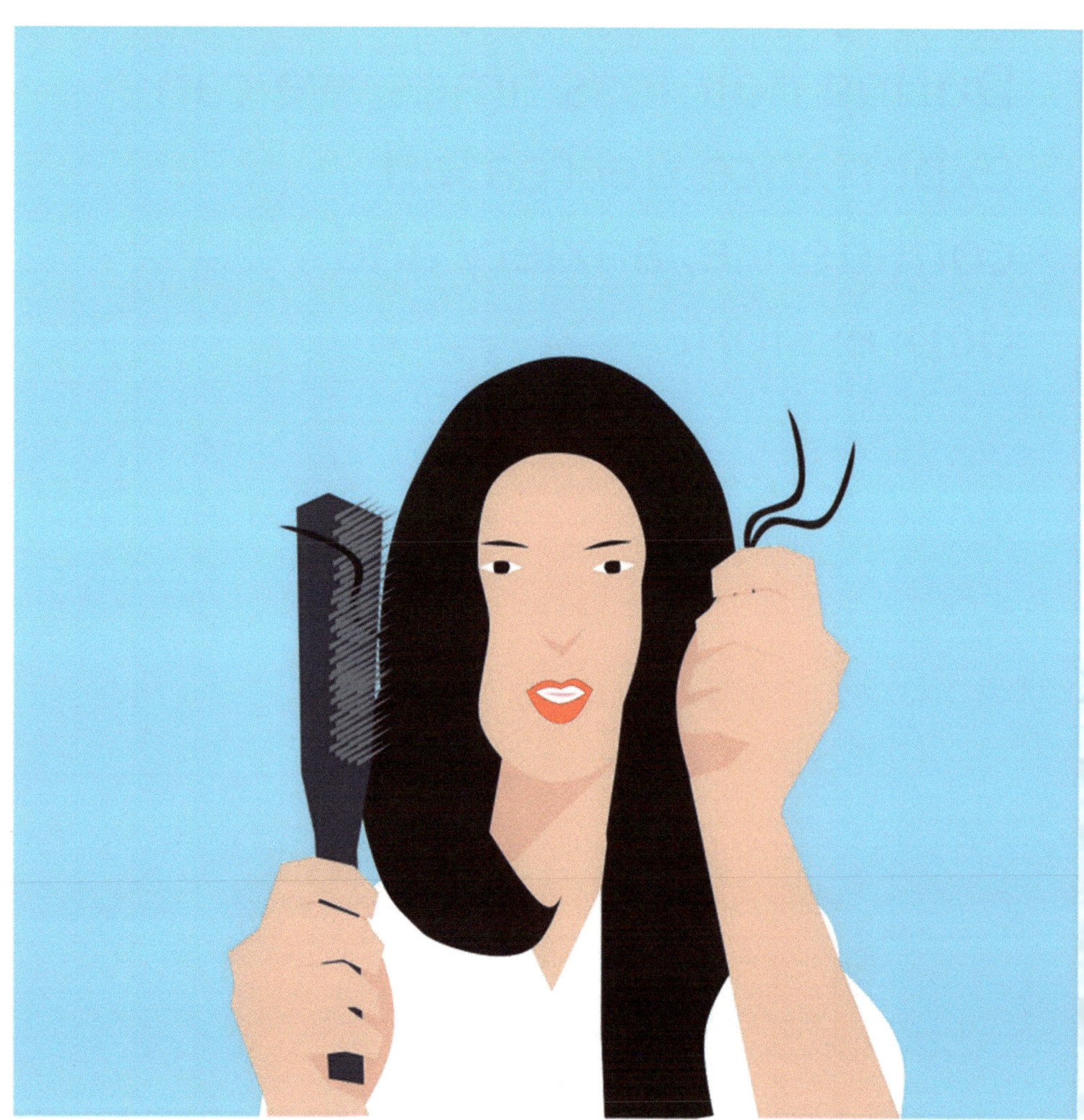

Studies have shown that hair loss has a negative psychological impact on a person's view of their body image, self-esteem and self confidence.

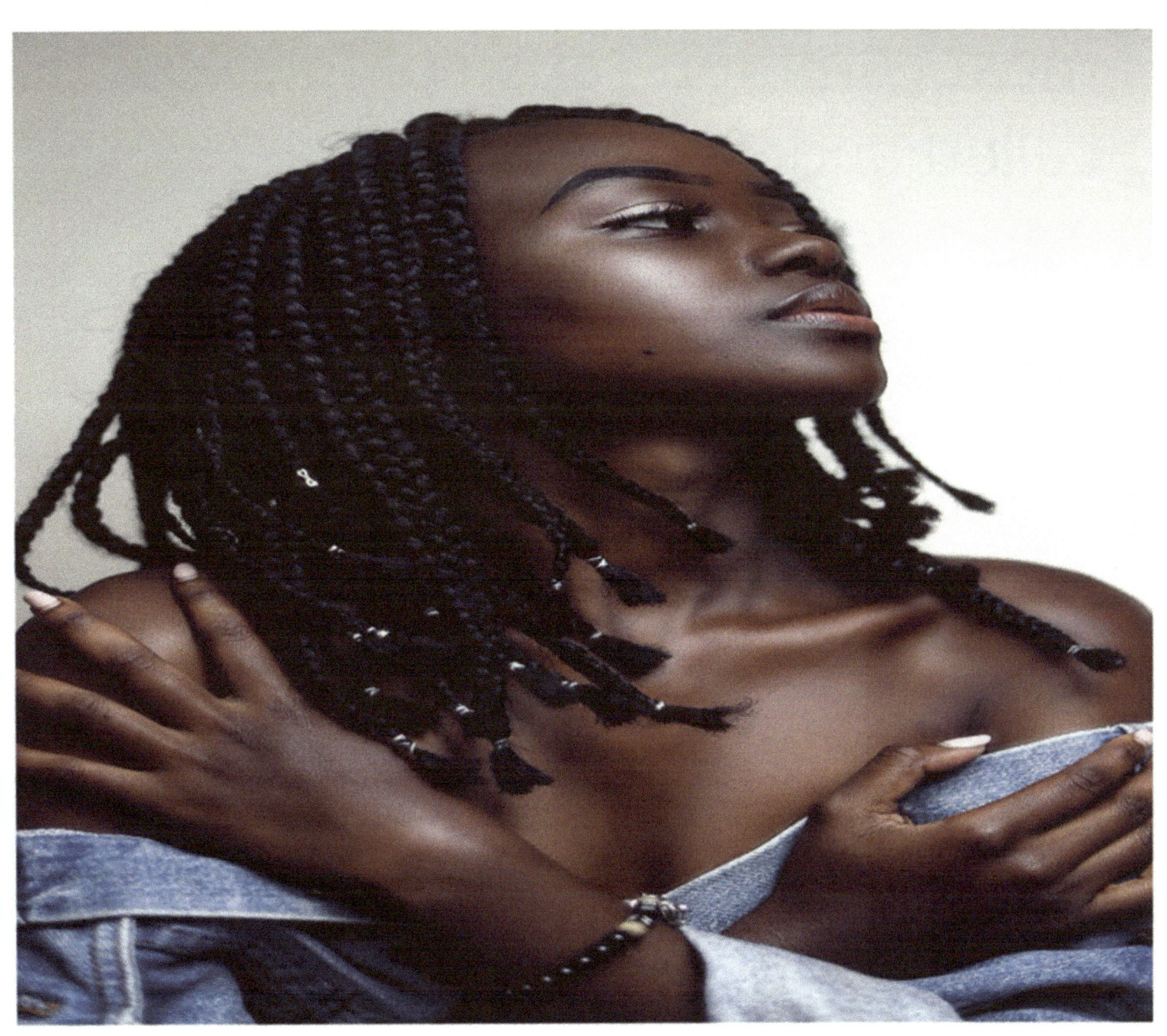

Love is patient and kind.
1 CORINTHIANS 13:4

Most all of us are familiar with the most common cause of hair loss called androgenic alopecia. Androgenic alopecia includes both male- and female-pattern baldness. It is hereditary, and its likelihood increases with age.

_____

_____

_____

_____

There are many reasons for hair loss. Some causes include pregnancy, thyroid conditions or anemia. There are other disorders, such as autoimmune diseases, psoriasis, seborrheic dermatitis, or polycystic ovary syndrome, that can cause hair loss, as well.

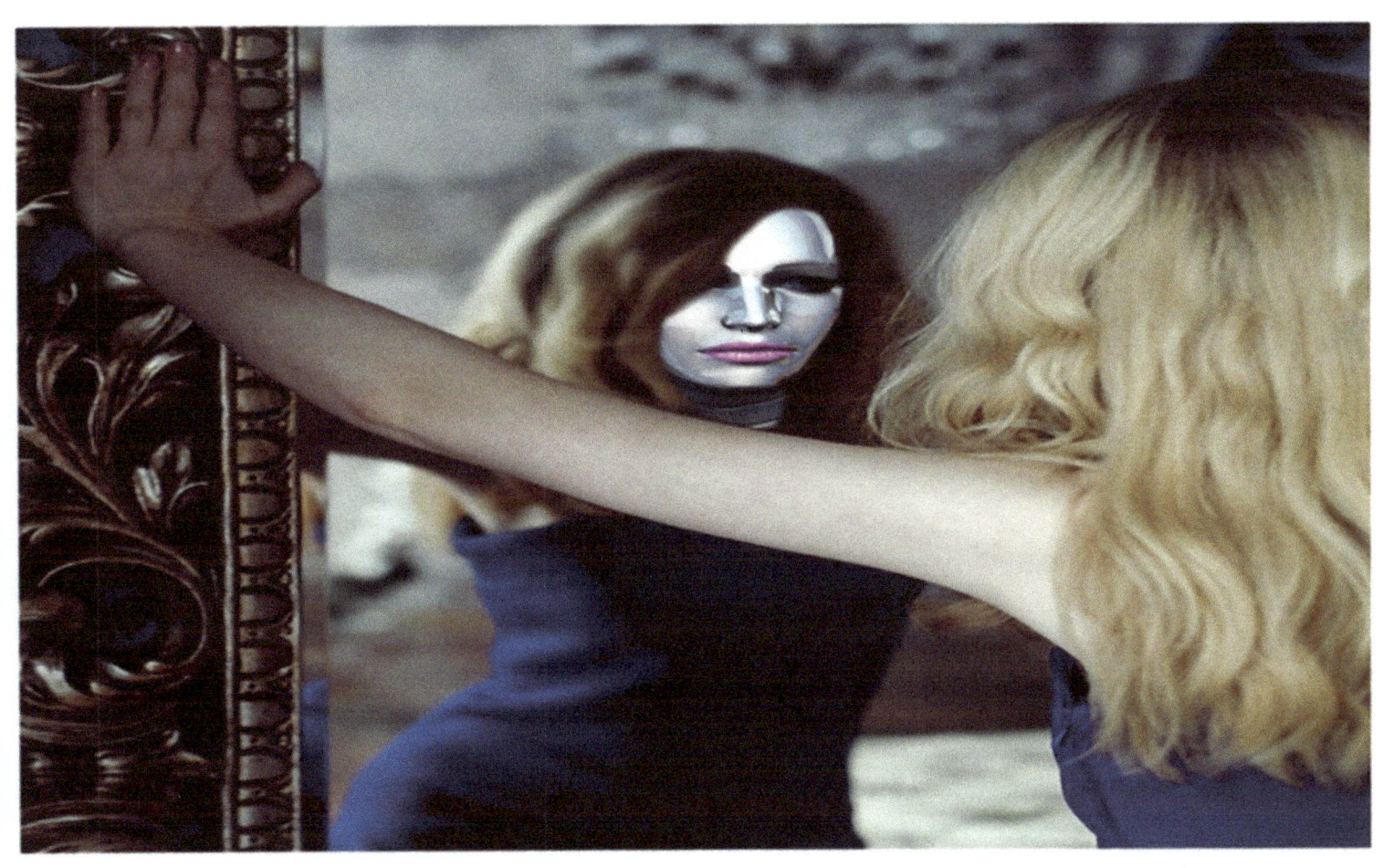

The three cycles of hair growth are anagen, catagen and telogen. Anagen is the growth phase lasting from two to eight years. About 90% of the hair on a head is in the Anagen Phase.

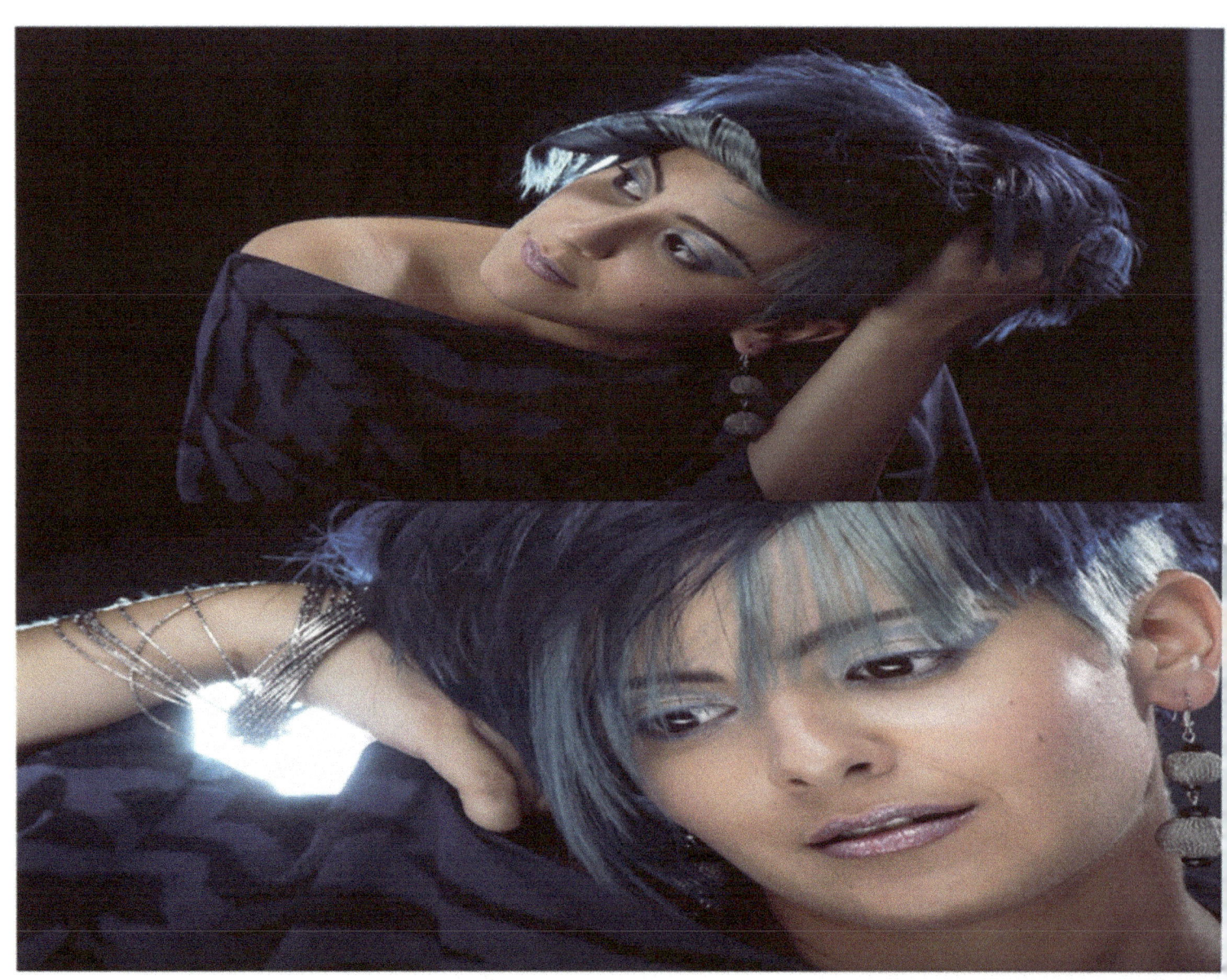

Catagen is the second phase, and it is the transition phase. This phase last about two to three weeks. The hair follicle shrinks during this time.

The third phase of hair growth is called the telogen cycle. This phase last about two to four months. This is when the hair is at rest. Yes, even the hair cycle must include rest. Did you know that your hair stops growing to rest? What do you think about that?

_____

_____

_____

For most people, hair grows about six inches a year. Normally, 10% of the hair strands on the head are in either transition or resting phases. This means the other 90% of the strands are growing.

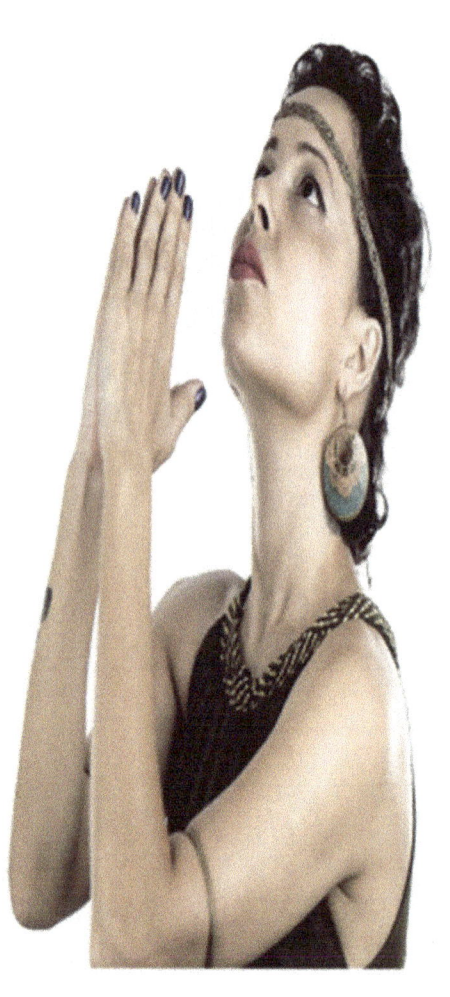

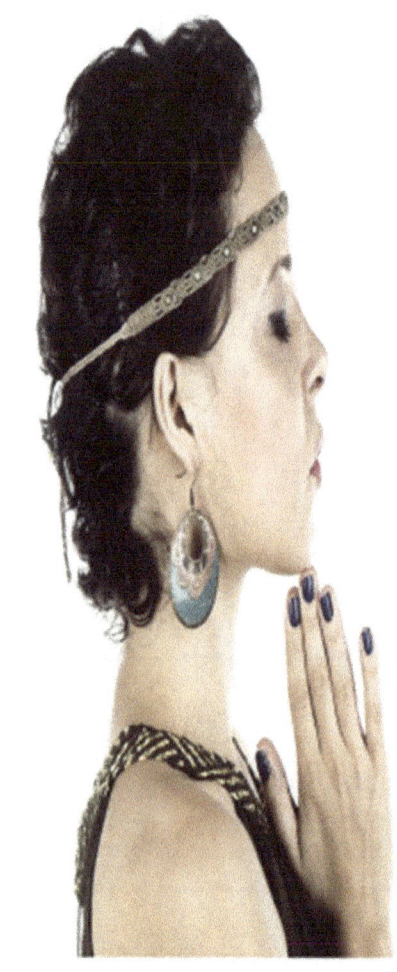

Guess what? Most people lose 50 to 100 strands of hair a day. However, during wash days, up to 250 strands of hair can be lost. Not to worry about that, because those stands were waiting to fall out. So continue to wash your hair!

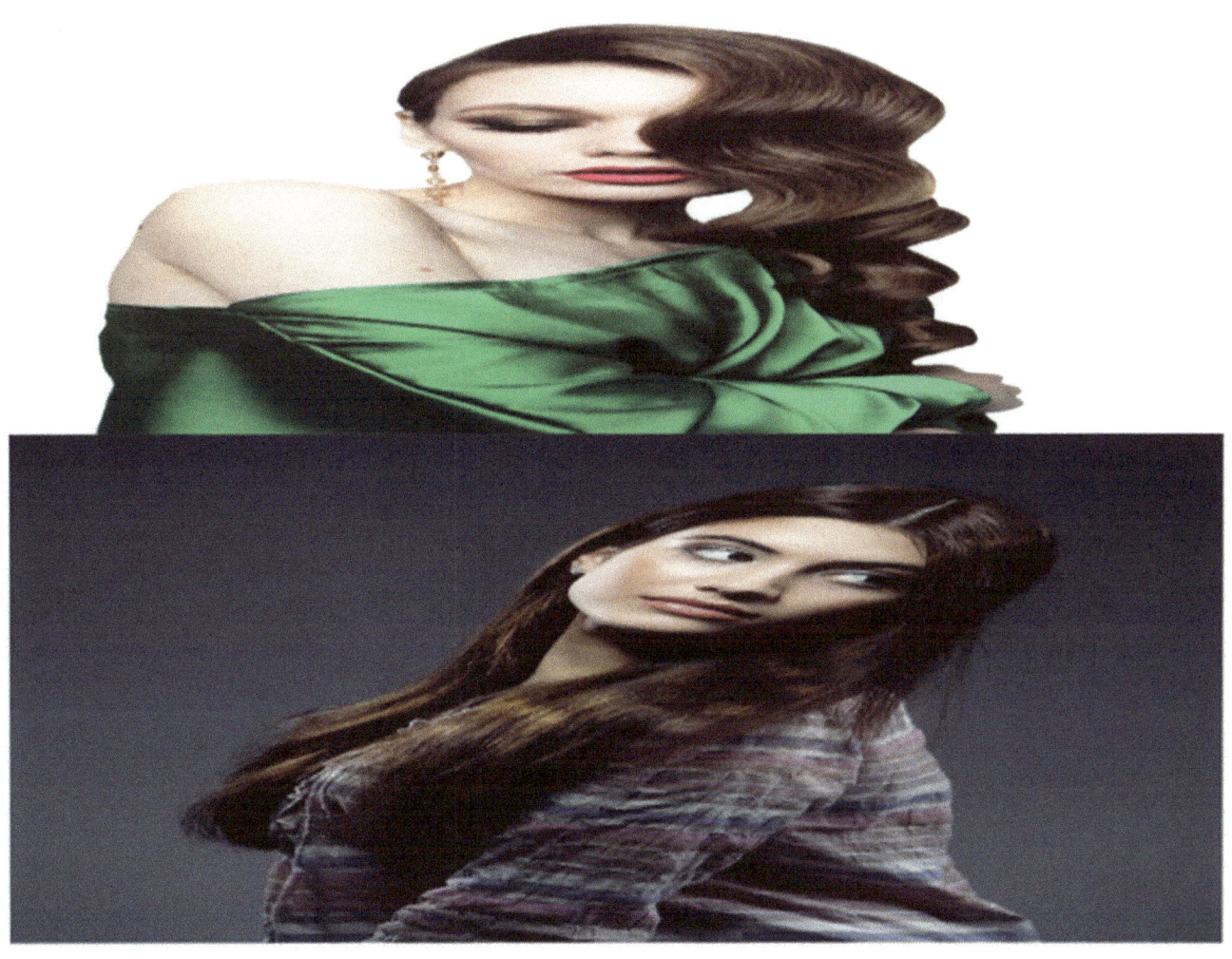

Gentle words are a tree of life; a deceitful tongue crushes the spirit.
PROVERBS 15: 4

Men's hair recedes from the forehead or crown of the head. Women tend to thin on the top third to one half of the scalp. They may also notice that their parts are getting wider.

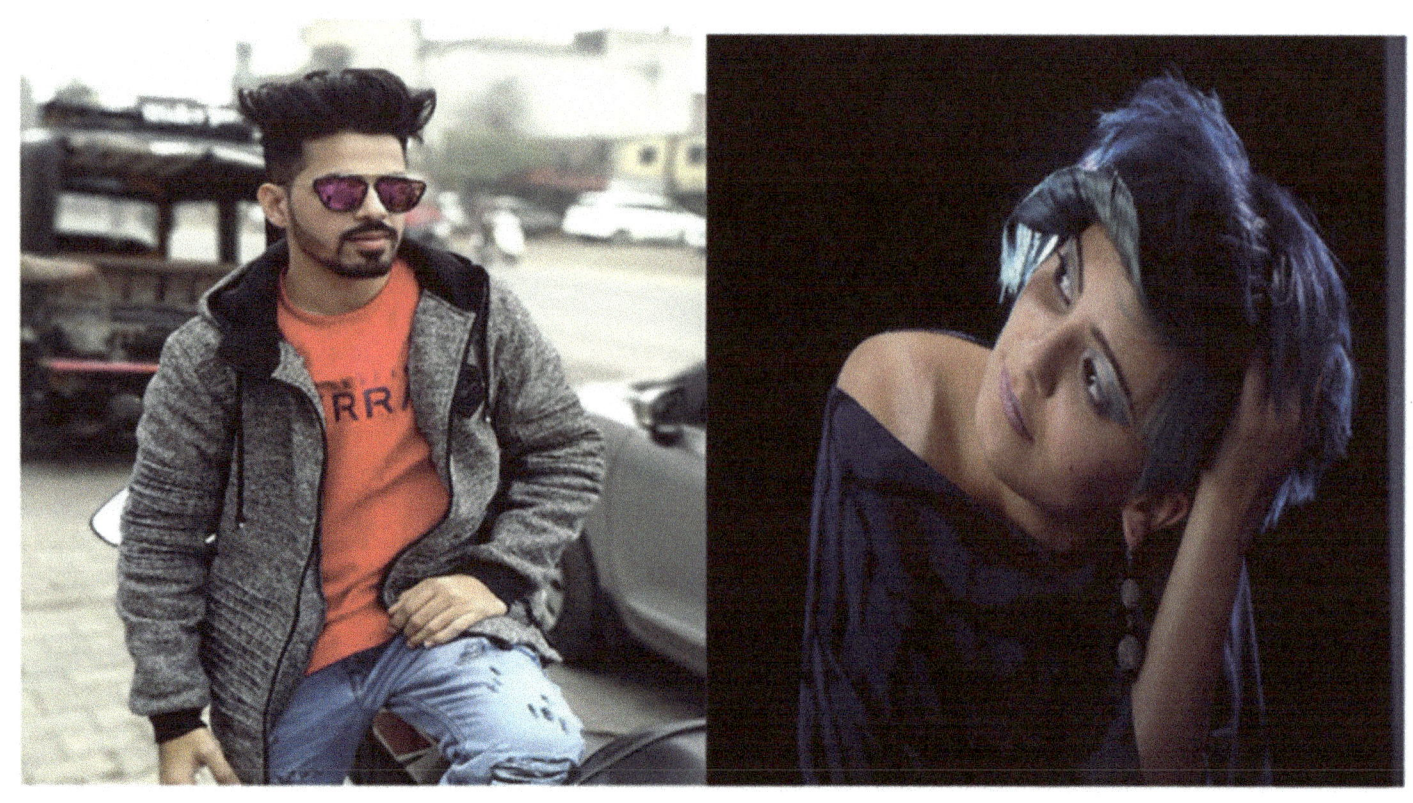

We will speak the truth in love, growing in every way more and more like Christ, who is the head of his body, the church.
EPHESIANS 4:15

If a grandmother, aunt, and mother all have the same amount of hair loss, this can be an indication of hair loss do to genetics. This is called, androgenetic alopecia.

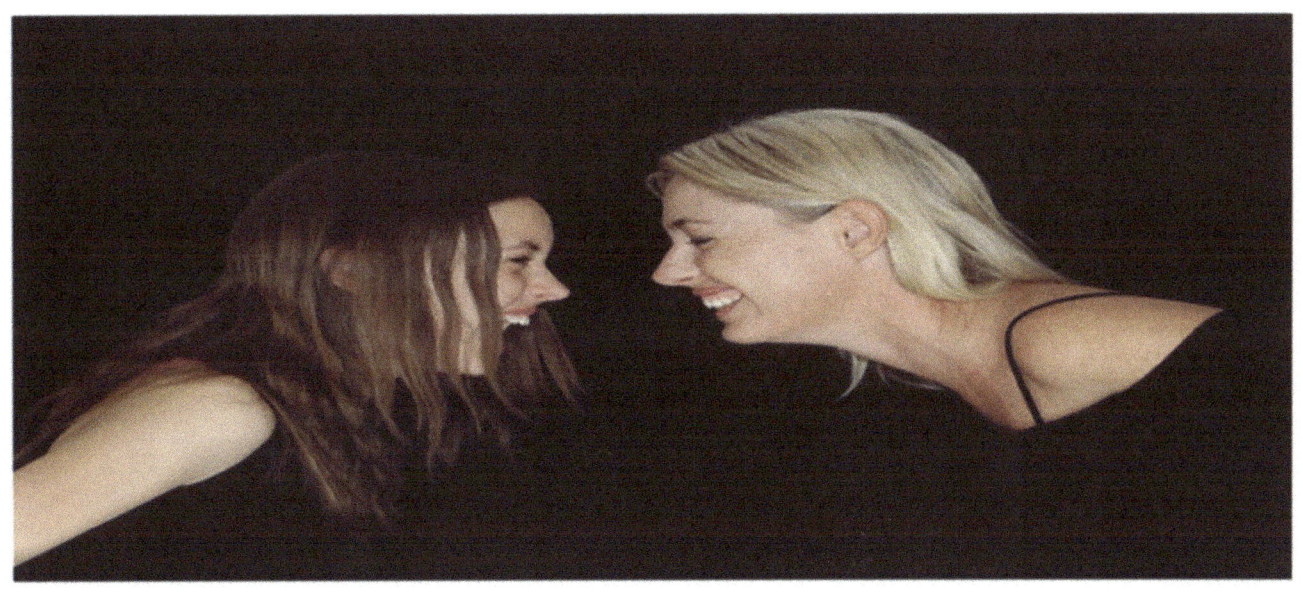

Alopecia Areata is a disease that develops when the body's immune system attacks hair follicles, causing hair loss.

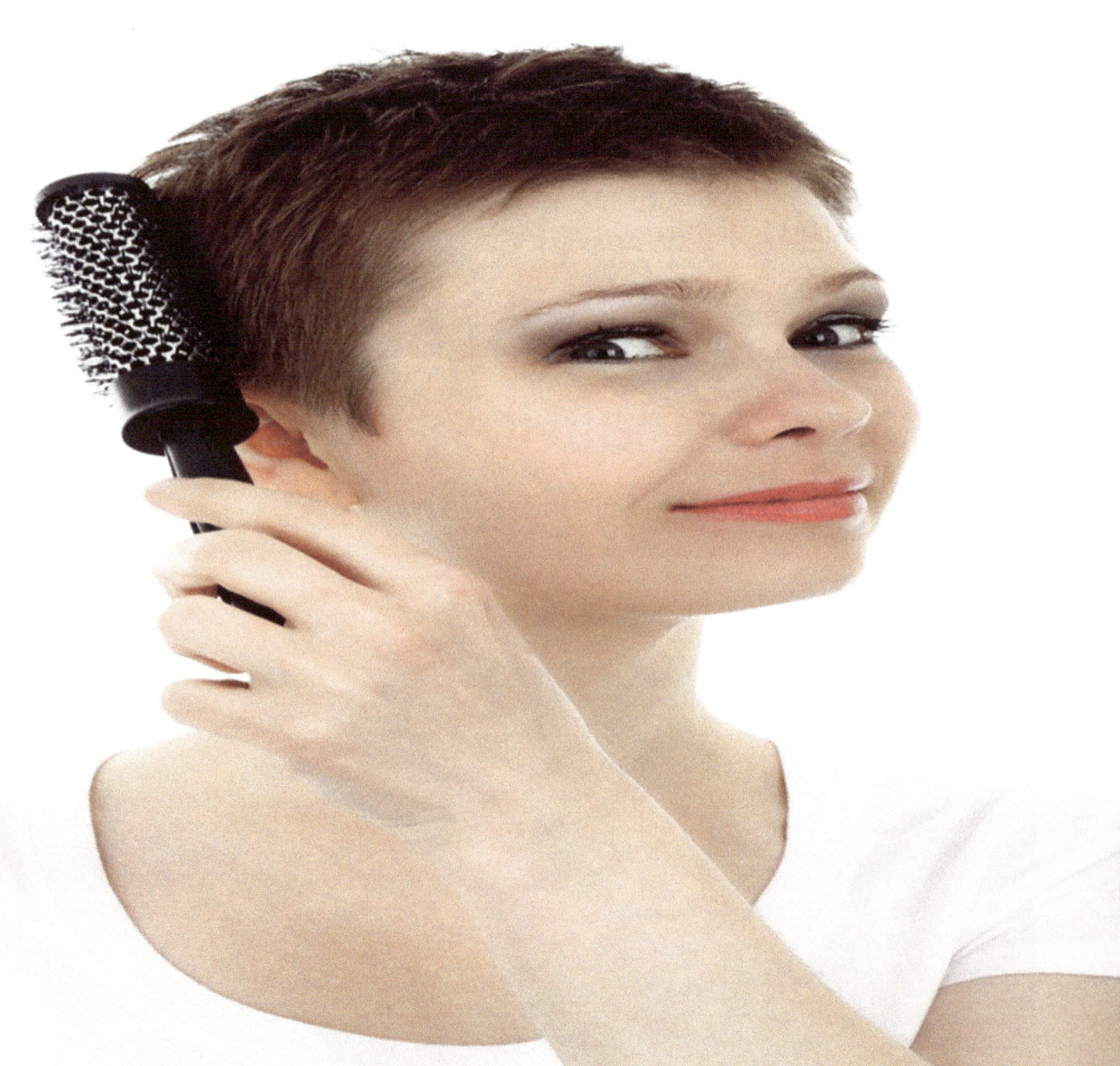

Polycystic ovary syndrome (PCOS) leads to cysts on a women's ovaries. Hormonal imbalances that result from this syndrome can cause hair loss.

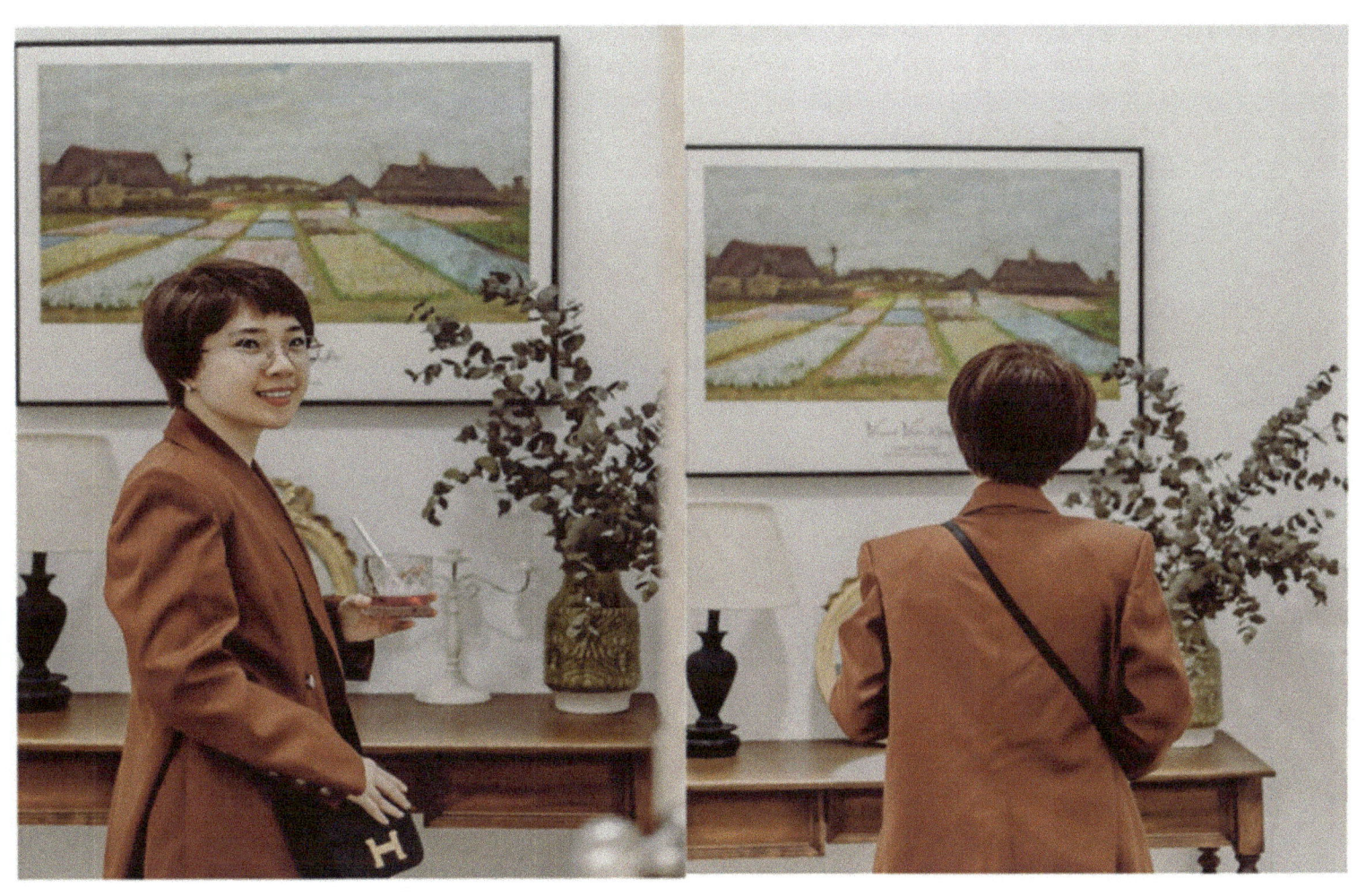

If you need wisdom, ask our generous God, and he will give it to you. He will not rebuke you for asking.
JAMES 1:5

A scalp infection can cause hair loss. When the infection clears, the hair will grow back.

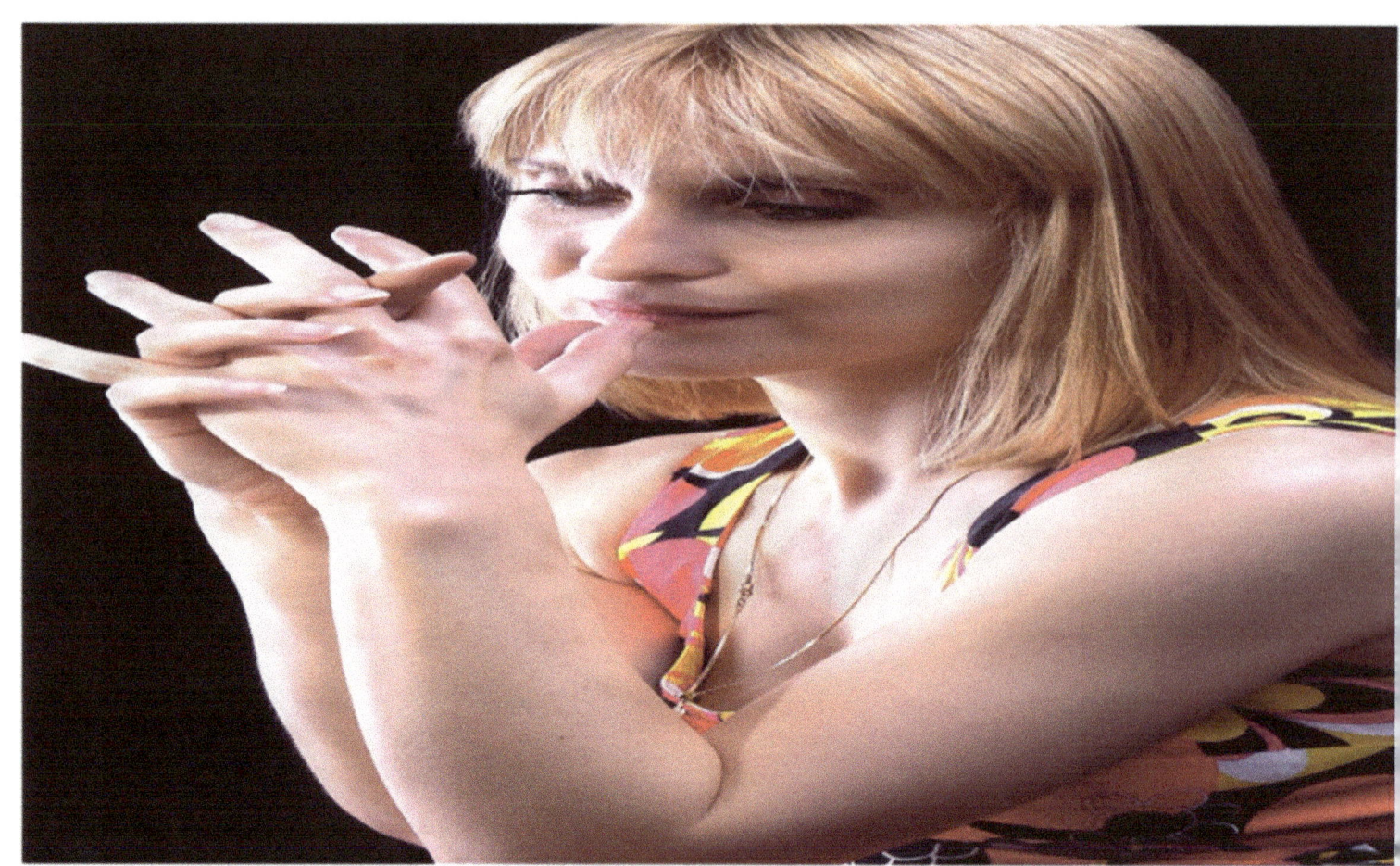

You, too, must be patient. Take courage, for the coming of the Lord is near.
JAMES 5: 8

Some medications will cause hair loss. Always check with your doctor before the discontinued use of your prescribed medications.

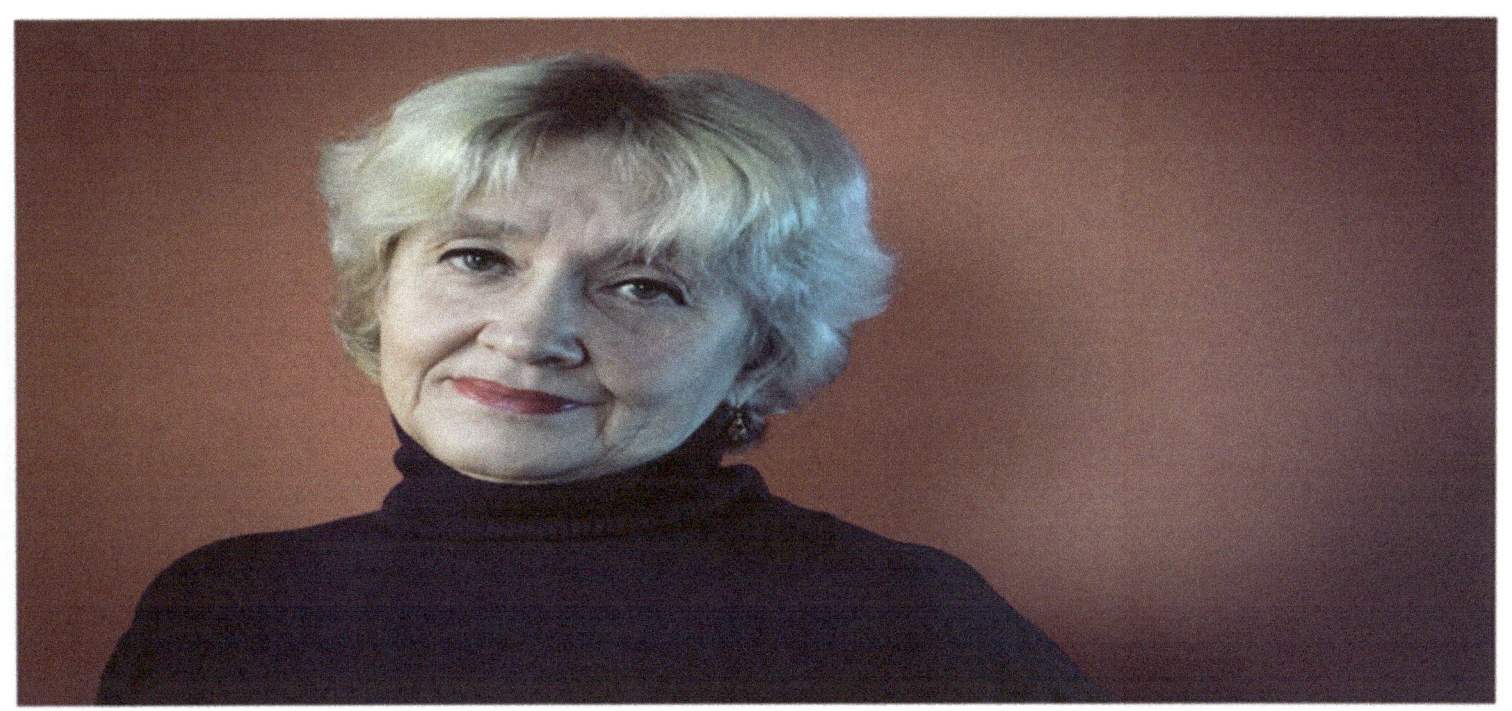

Scarring Alopecia can cause hair loss. After a hair follicle has been distroyed, the hair will no longer grow from that follicle. The most common cause of scarring alopecia is from inflammation.

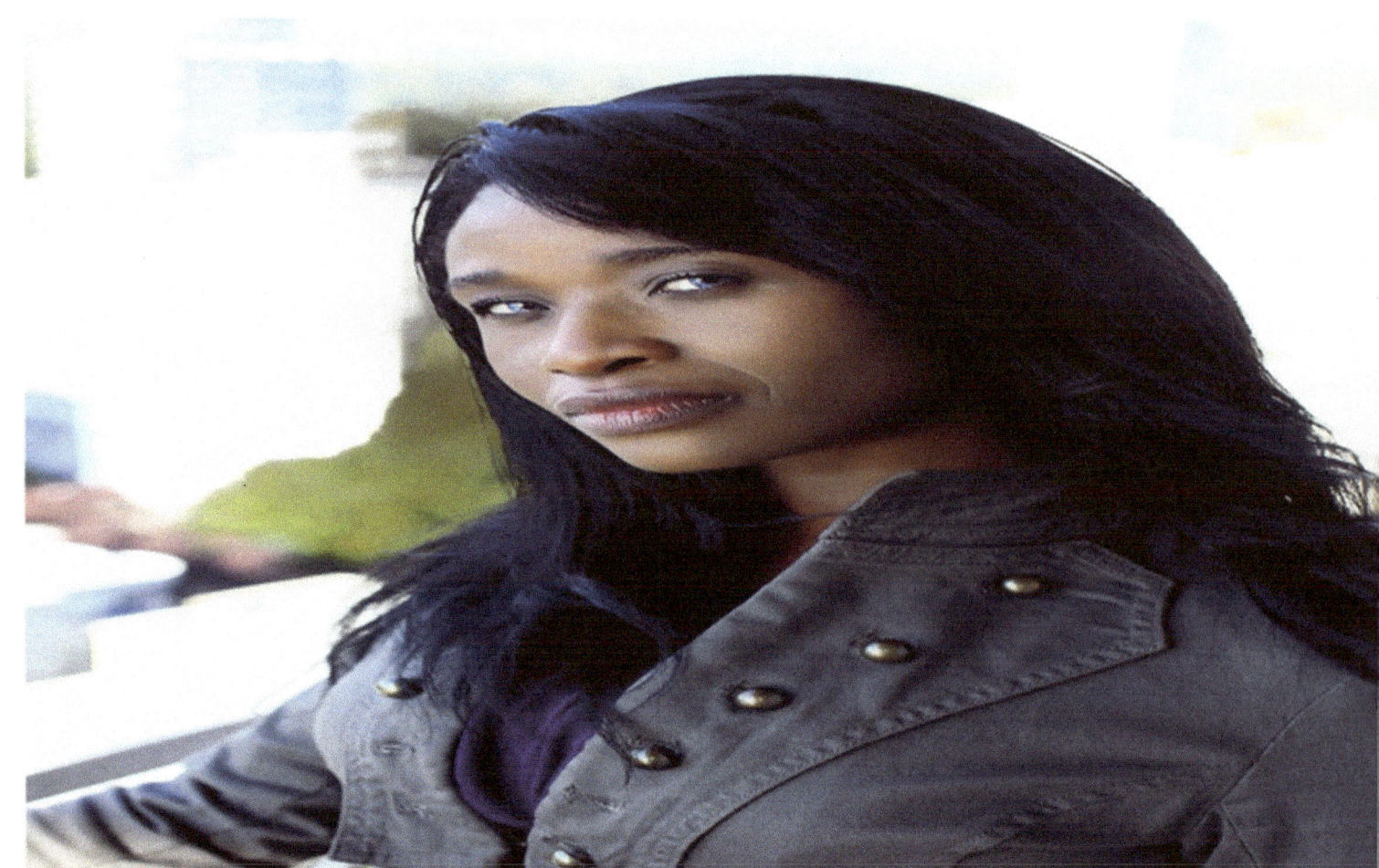

Take your vitamins. If your body is lacking one or more necessary nutrients, such as biotin, iron, protein or zinc, you can experience hair loss. Once your body gets suffecient nutricion, the hair will grow back.

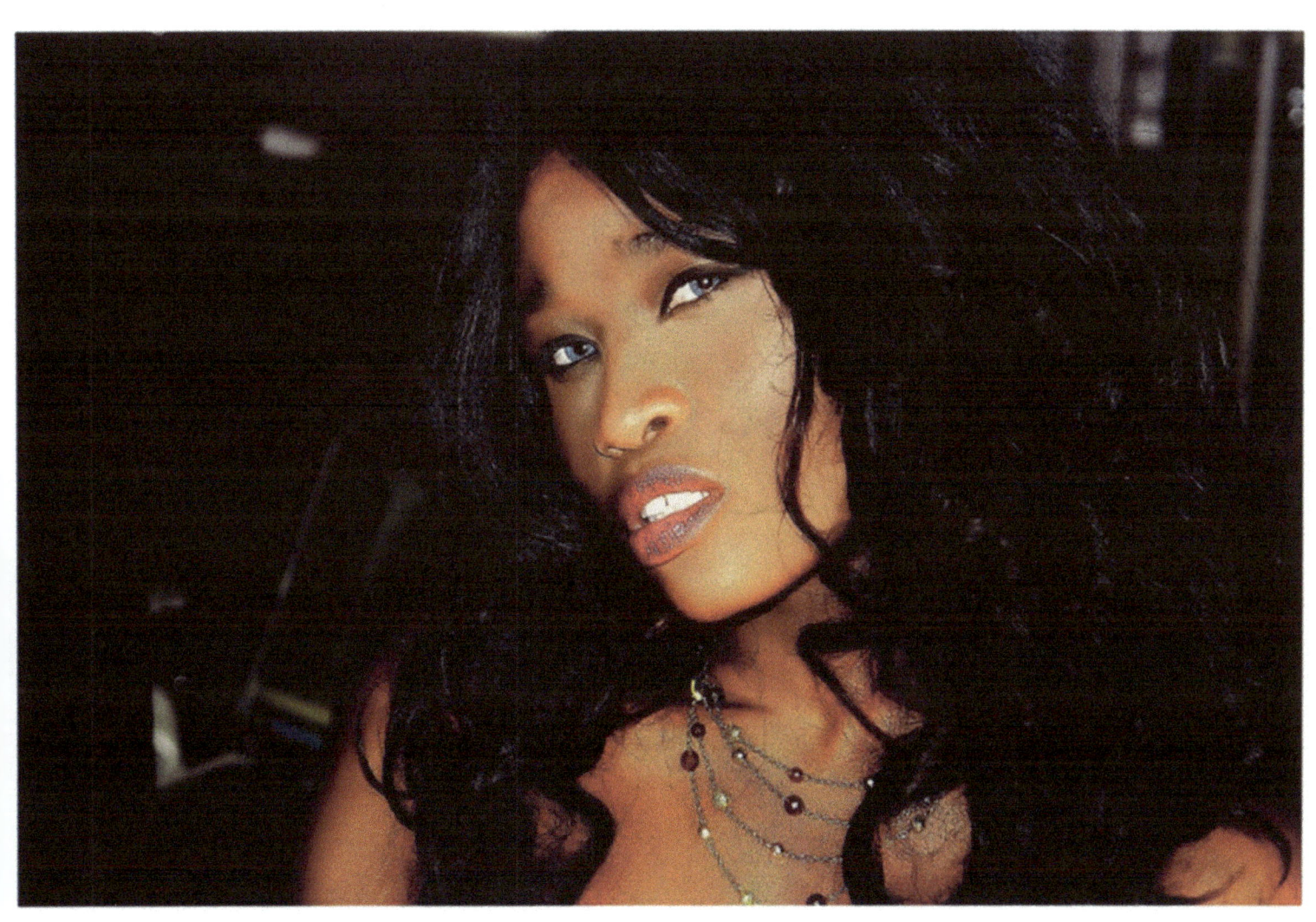

Those who are peacemakers will plant seeds of peace and reap a harvest of righteousness.
JAMES 3:18

The continual pulling of hair or wearing your hair too tight can lead to permanent hair loss called traction alopecia.

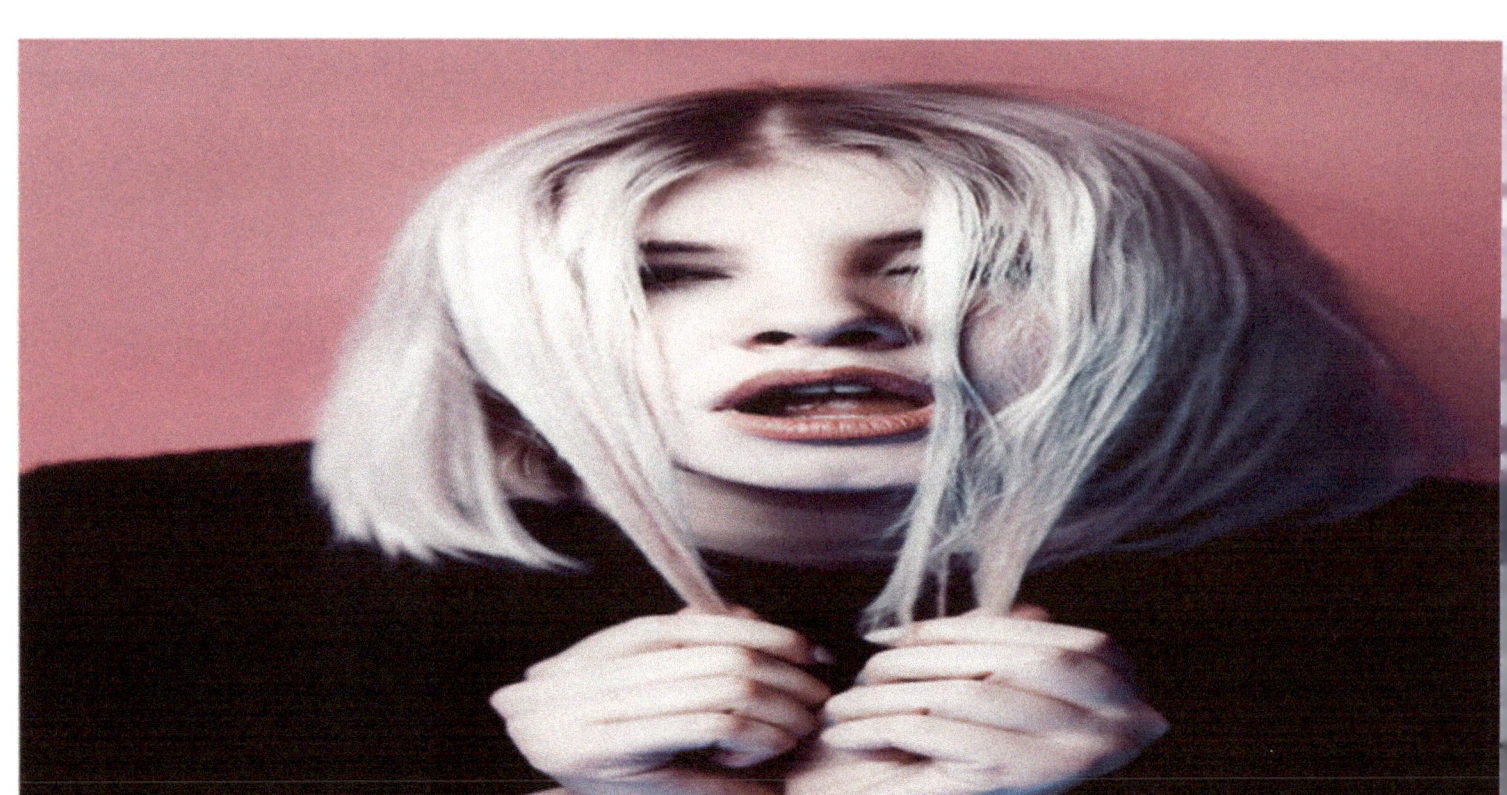

Focal loss is when your hair loss appears in patches on the body or scalp. It is an autoimmune disorder that mostly develops in early childhood. However, it can affect people of all ages, sexes, race, or ethnicities.

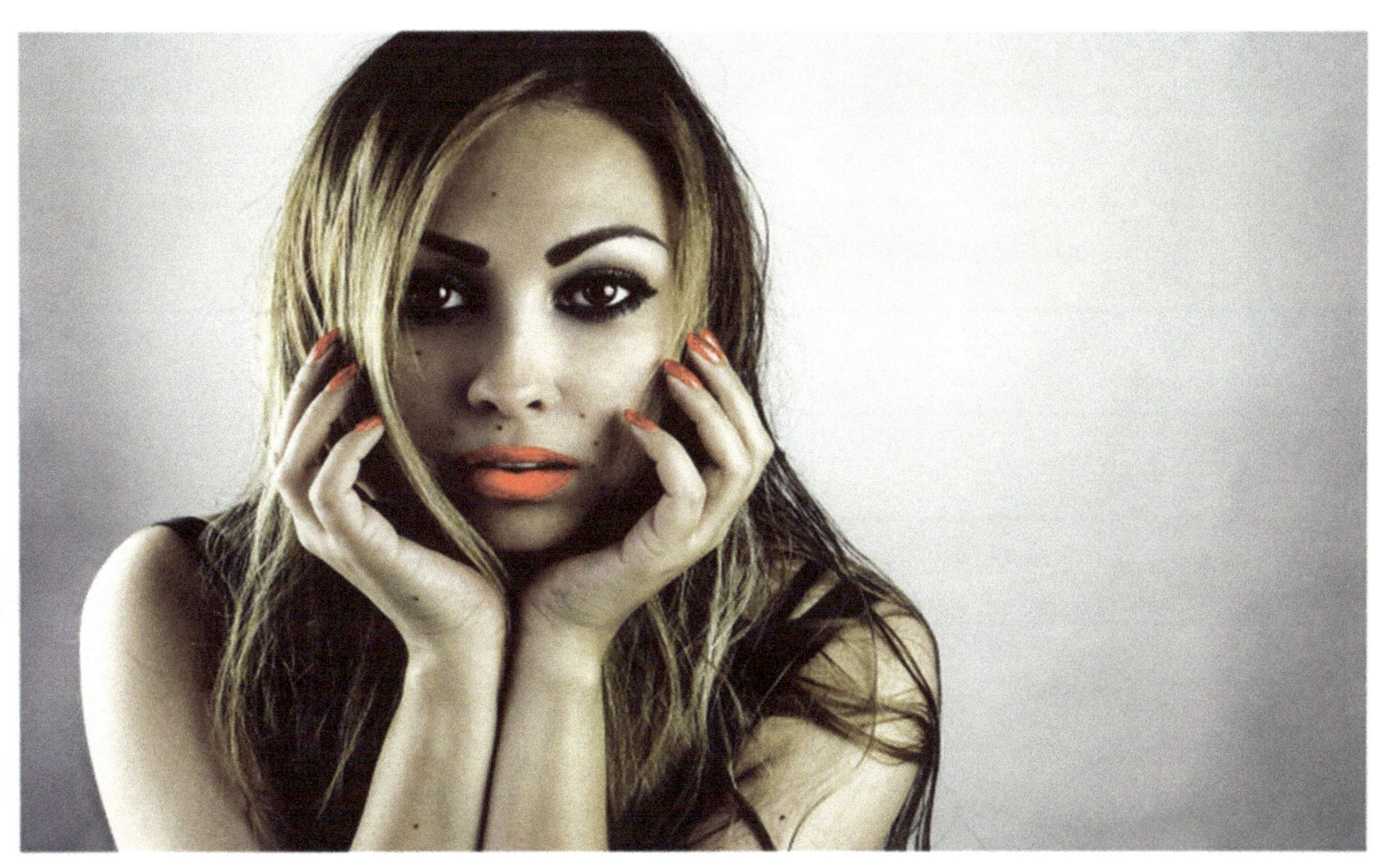

We know that God causes everything to work together for the good of those who love God and are called according to his purpose for them.
ROMANS 8:28

When did you first notice your hair loss?

_____

_____

_____

_____

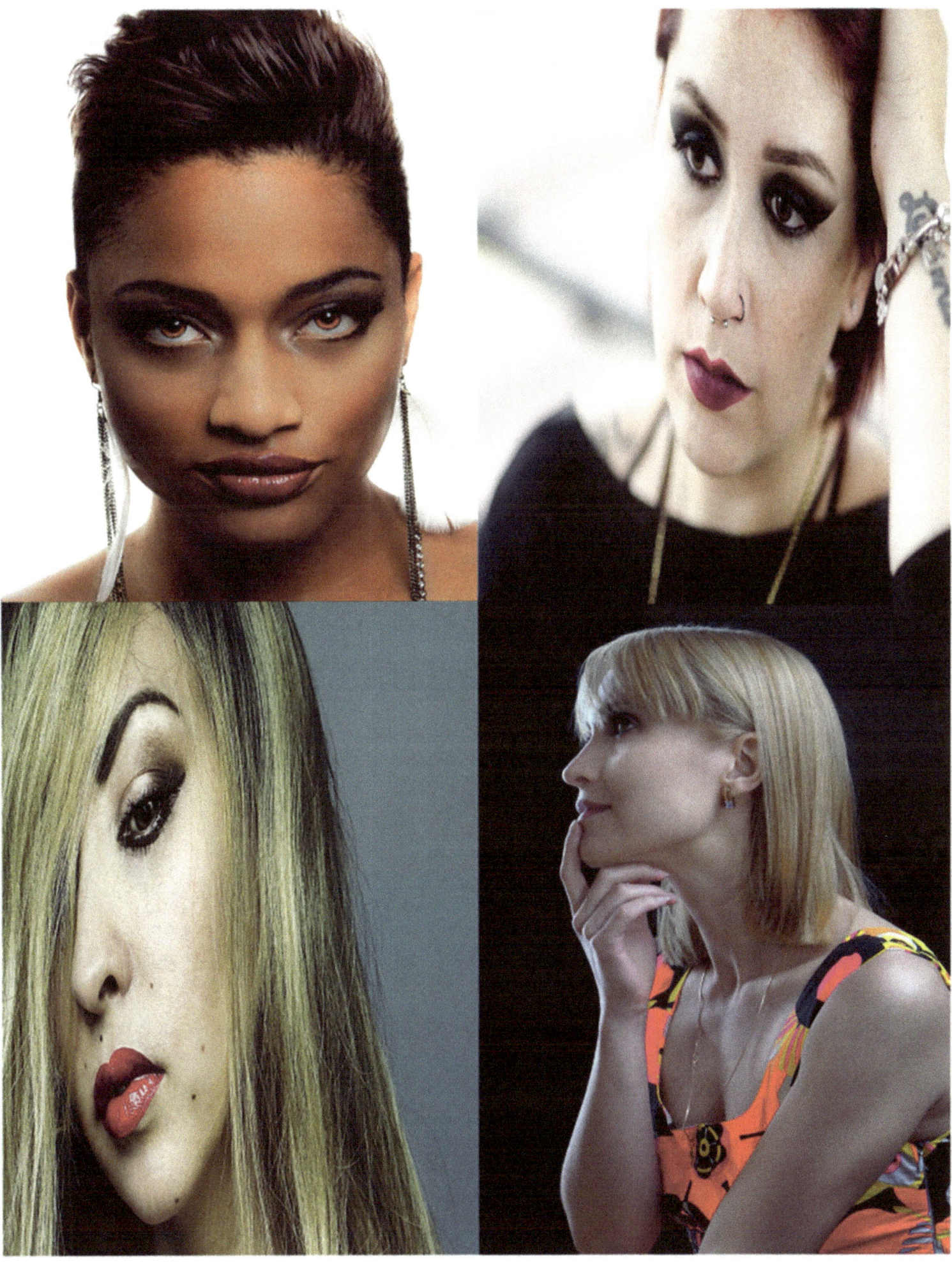

Praise the Lord; praise God our savior! For each day he carries us in his arms.   PSALM 68:19

Some medications may offer some solutions to hair loss, including minoxidil, corticosteroids, finasteride, spironolactone, dutasteride, and others. Be aware that these medications have various side affects and may or may not be helpful to your hair growth journey. Do some research and talk with your doctor about any medications that you may consider using.

Documement the results of any medications that you are using. Did any hair grow back? How long did it take to see progress of hair growth? Did you experience any side effects while taking the medication?

_____

_____

_____

_____

_____

_____

_____

_____

You never have to be alone on your hair loss journey. There are over 80 million people in America suffering from hair loss. Thirty percent of men lose their hair by the age of 35. Forty percent of people that loose hair are women. So many people lose hair that the month of August has been declared Hair Loss Awareness Month.

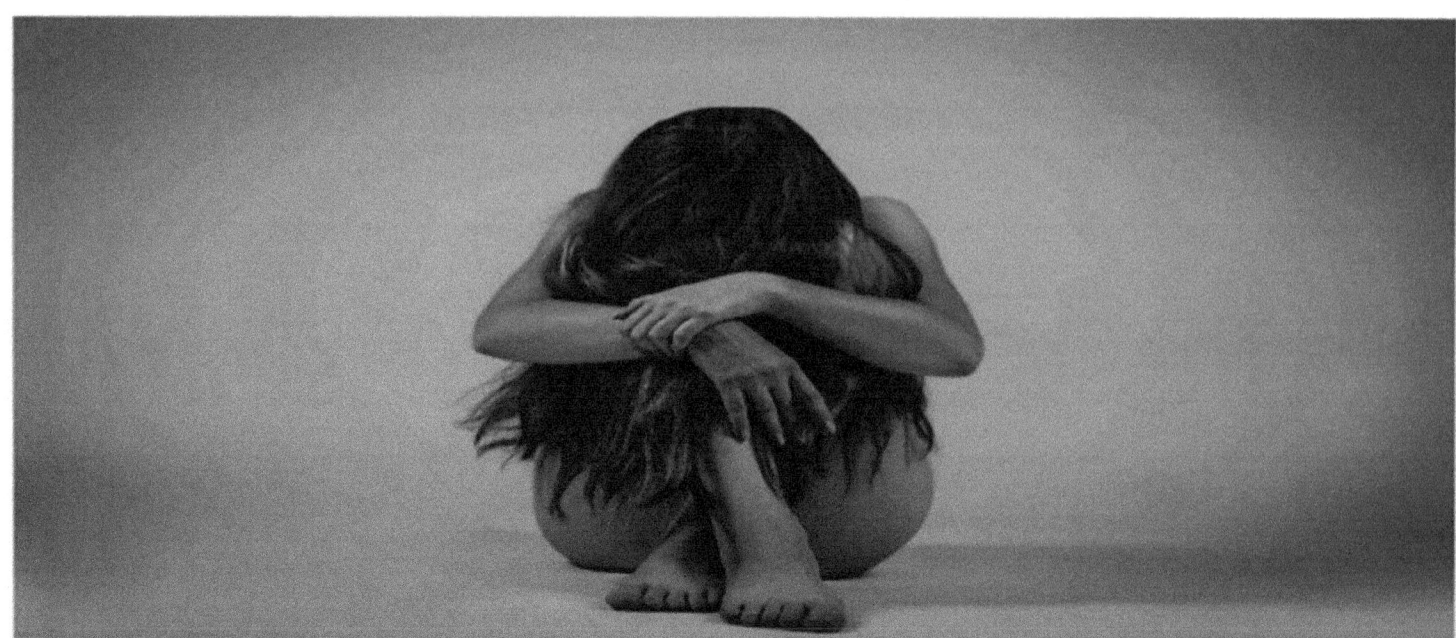

"Do not worry about it!" This is easier said, than done, right? We all understand that not worrying about hair loss is almost impossible to do. For some people, hair is a constant worry.

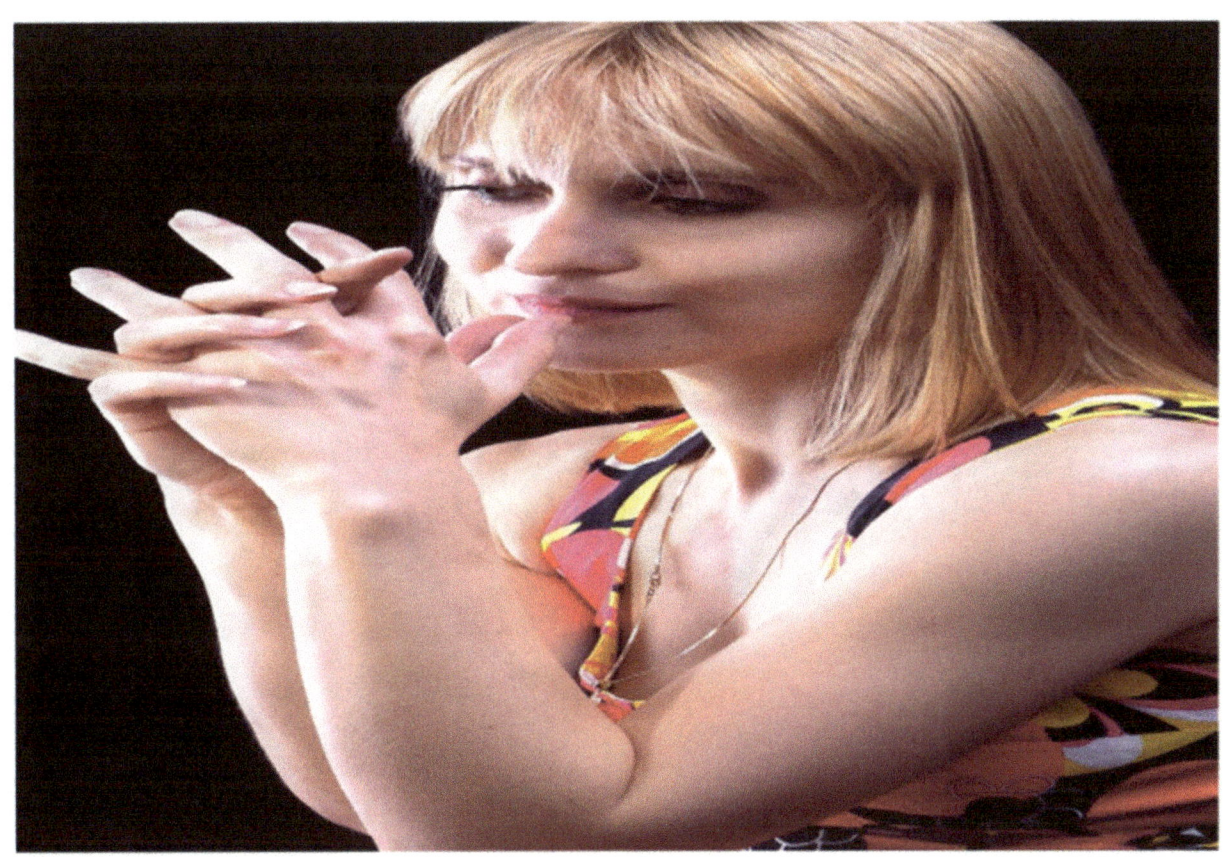

The blameless will be rescued from harm, but the crooked will be suddenly destroyed.
PROVERBS 28:18

This is a good time to share your fears about your hair loss. What are your thoughts concerning your loss? Who or what intimidates you about losing your hair? (For instance, one of my customer's concerns had to do with her high school students judging her.)

Do not lose confidence in your worth. Keep it all together. Remember that you are more than just your hair. Try new things that may inspire you. Practice self-care. Get out into nature and love on yourself always.

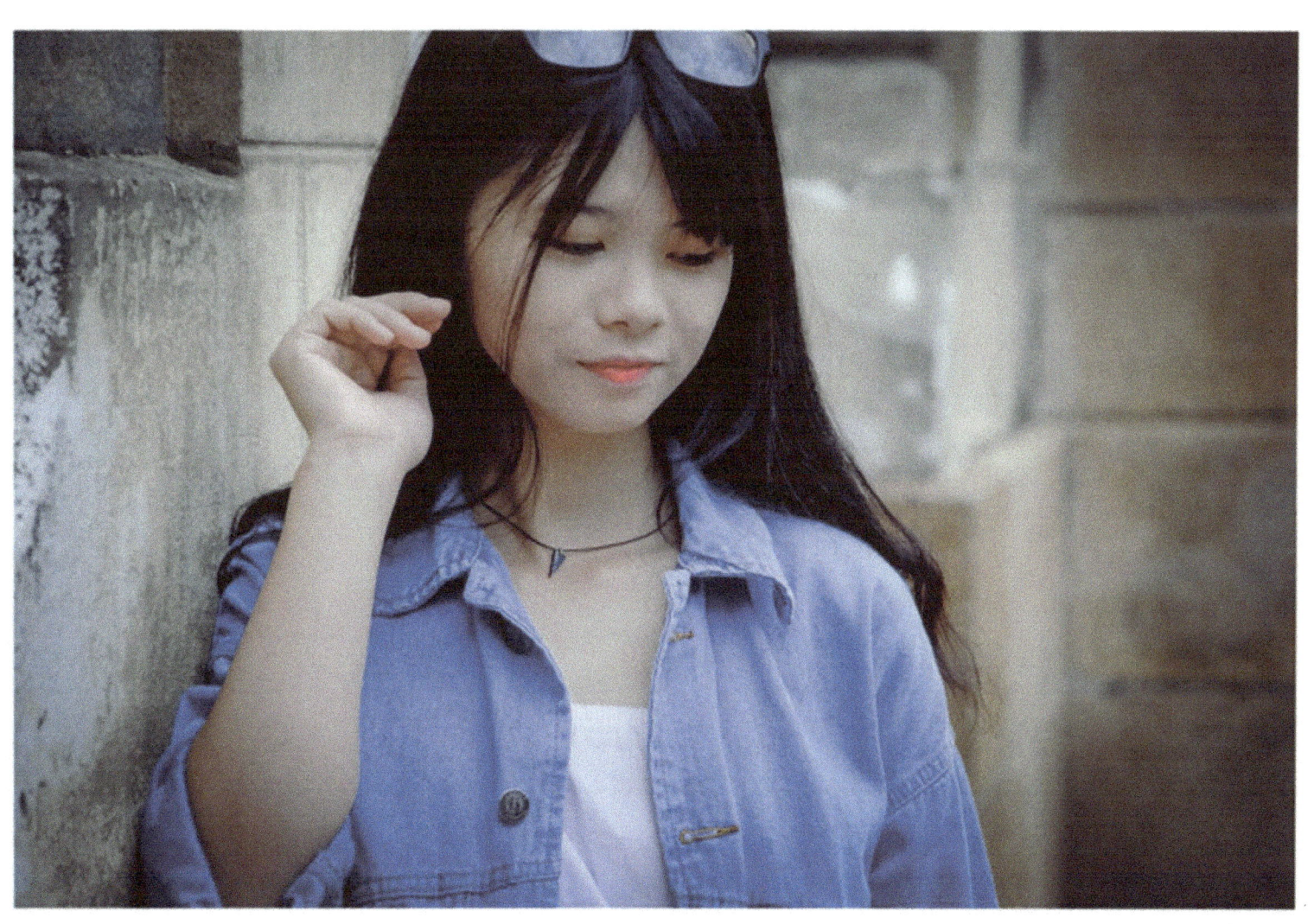

Let's not get tired of doing what is good. At just the right time we will reap a harvest of blessing if we don't give up.
GALATIANS 6:9

How are you feeling about yourself? Have you given up on being happy due to your hair loss?

Journel it out. Get a clear mind about how you are feeling.

_____

_____

Story Time...

I own a wig store serving the community of wig wearers. I get to hear many stories from people with hair loss issues. One story in particular is of a young lady who lost her hair because of an unusual occurrence. She shared with me that her boyfriend had cut her hair off while she was sleeping. He told her that short hair would make her less attractive. I was not anticipating such a story. However, it was a traumatic experience for her. I fit her for a wig and she regained her confidence.

It is true: for many of us, our hair is tied into our self-esteem and how we feel about ourselves. We make better decisions when we feel good about ourselves. We work harder, play harder, and take pride in our strengths.

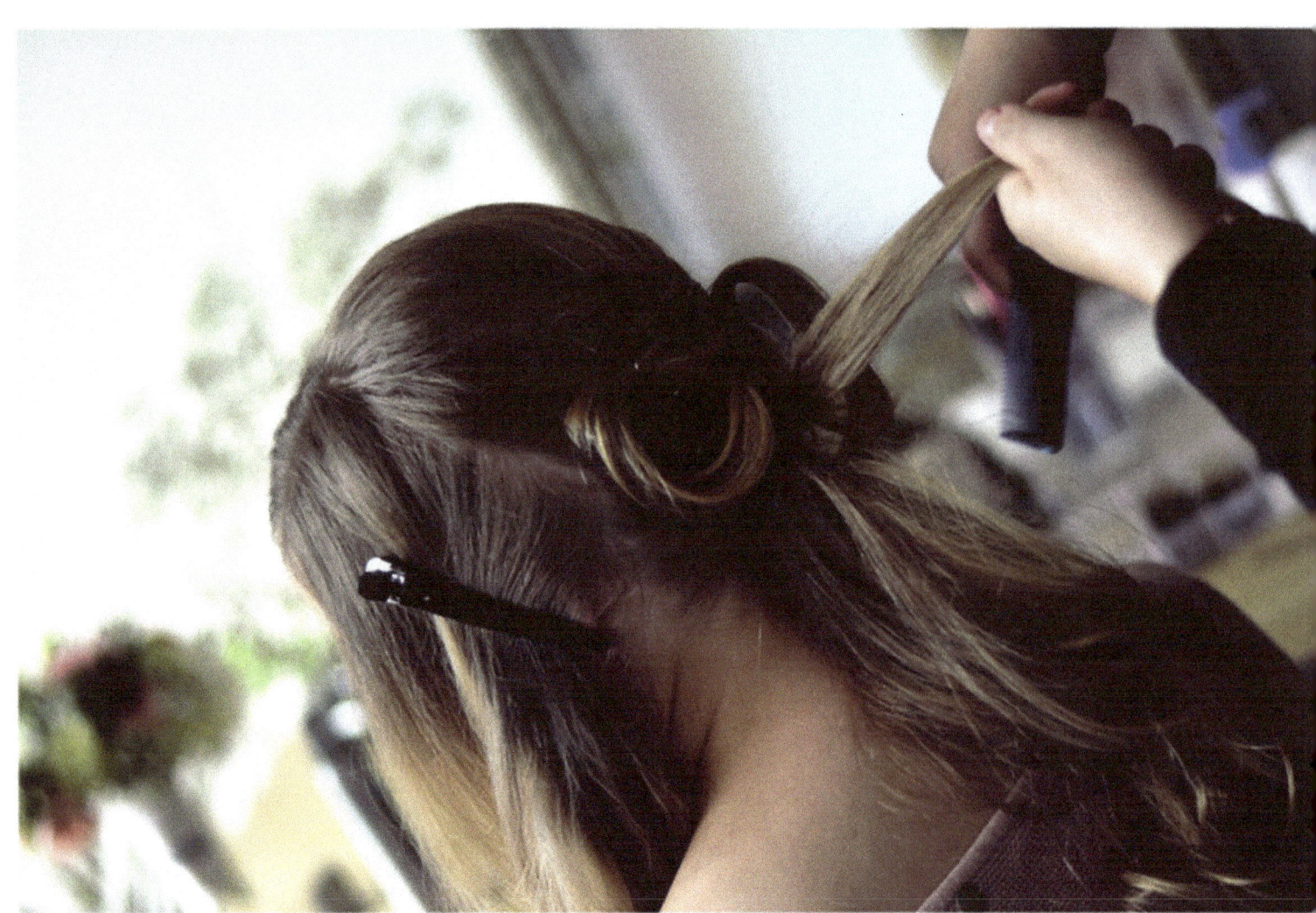

However, we all must remember that self-worth means that we value ourselves. We are worthy. You are worthy! You are a good person who deserves to be treated with respect. Know that you have value, are loveable, and are necessary to life. Therefore, your self-worth trumps your hair loss. Remember that you are most worthy! Can you address your worth? Think about your self-worth and journal your thoughts.

_____

_____

The Lord God is our sun and our shield. He gives us grace and glory. The Lord will withhold no good thing from those who do what is right.
PSALM 84: 11

Self check... Is your self-worth at the core of your very self? Your thoughts, feelings, and behaviors are at the root of how you view your worthiness and value as a person.

_____

_____

_____

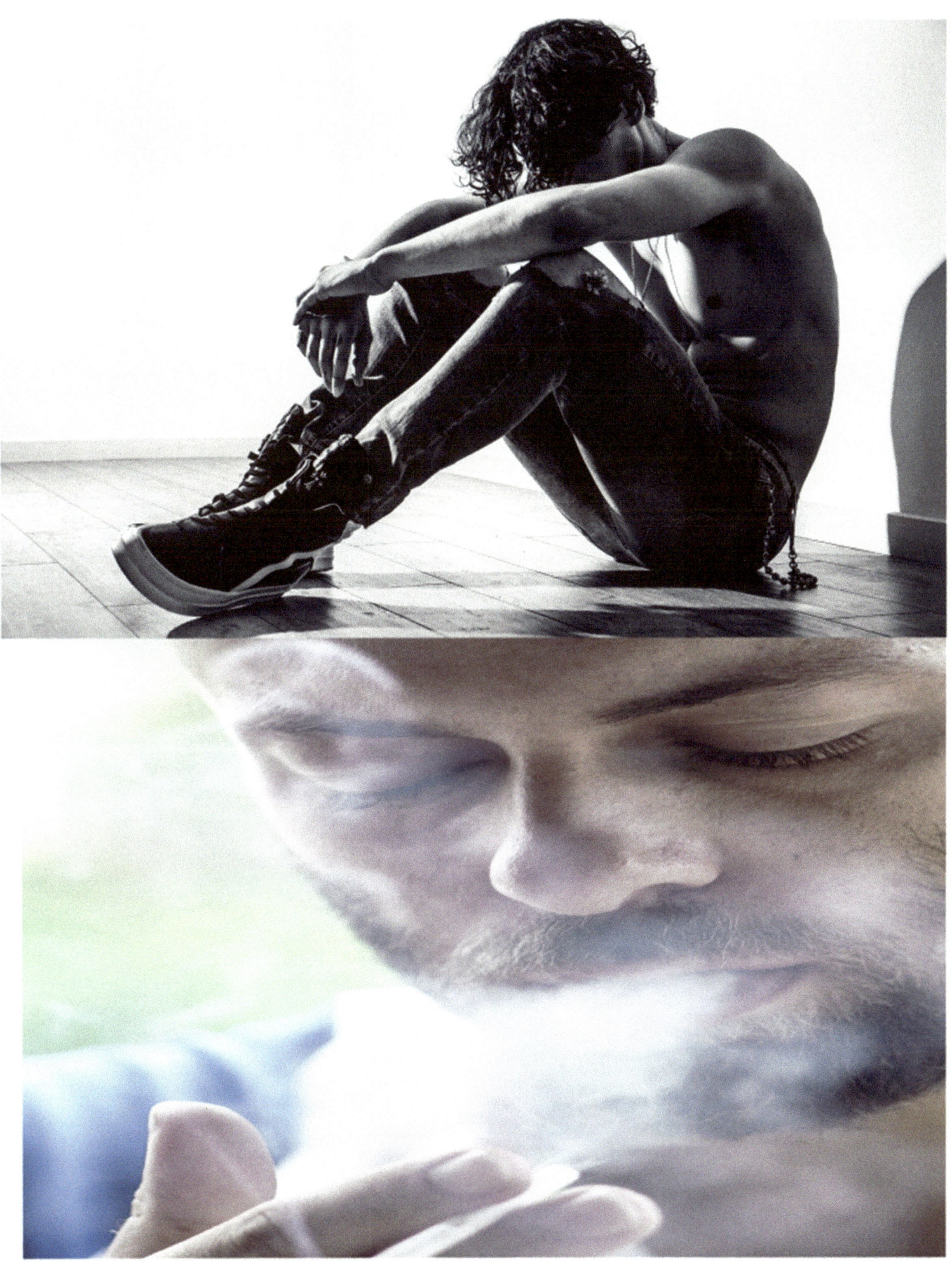

Take life by the hand and embrace a new quality of life. Learn from your experiences and share them with those whom may need your wisdom and knowledge. With, or without hair, you matter!

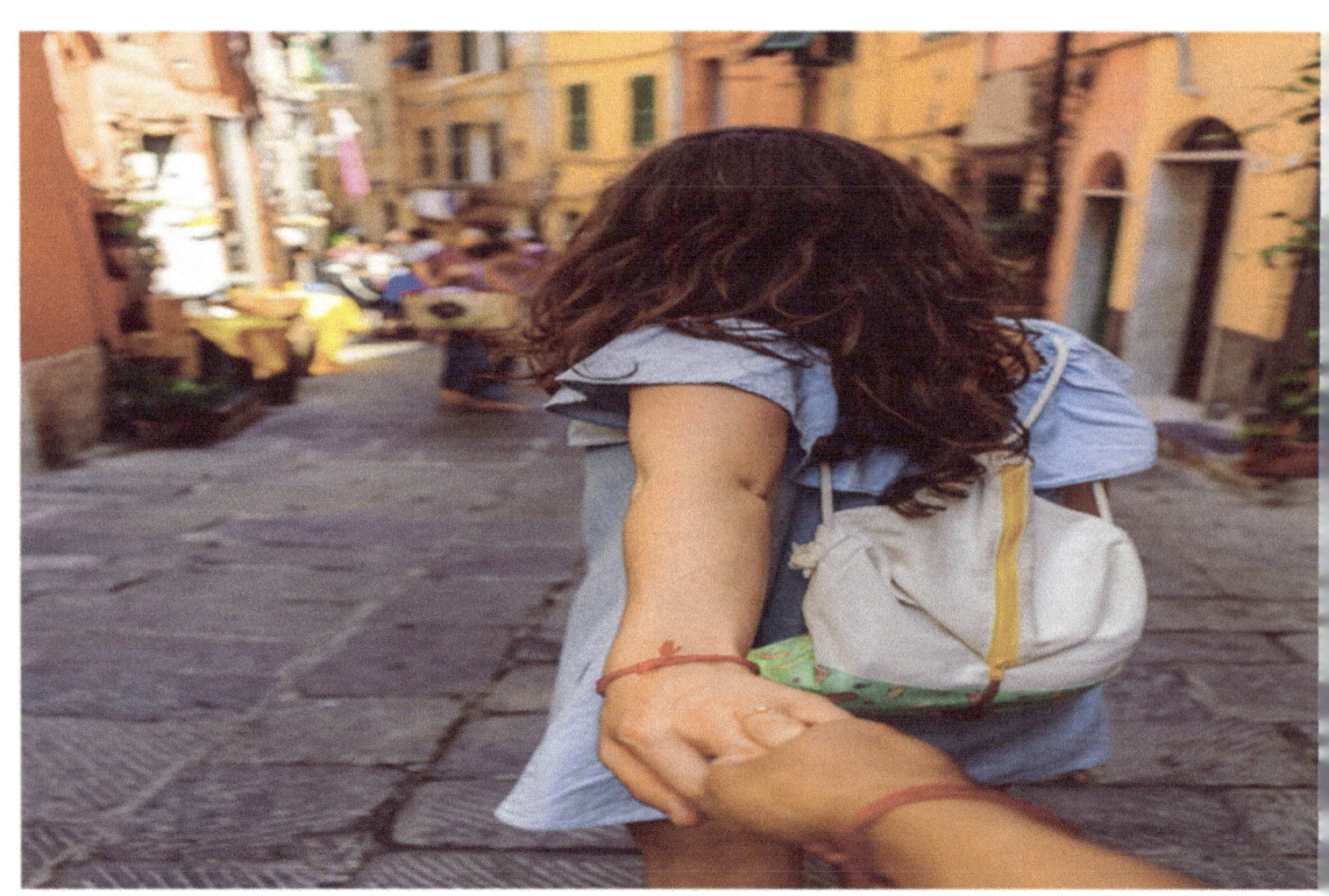

You are an awesome person. You will rise above any and all negative thoughts, or feelings about yourself.

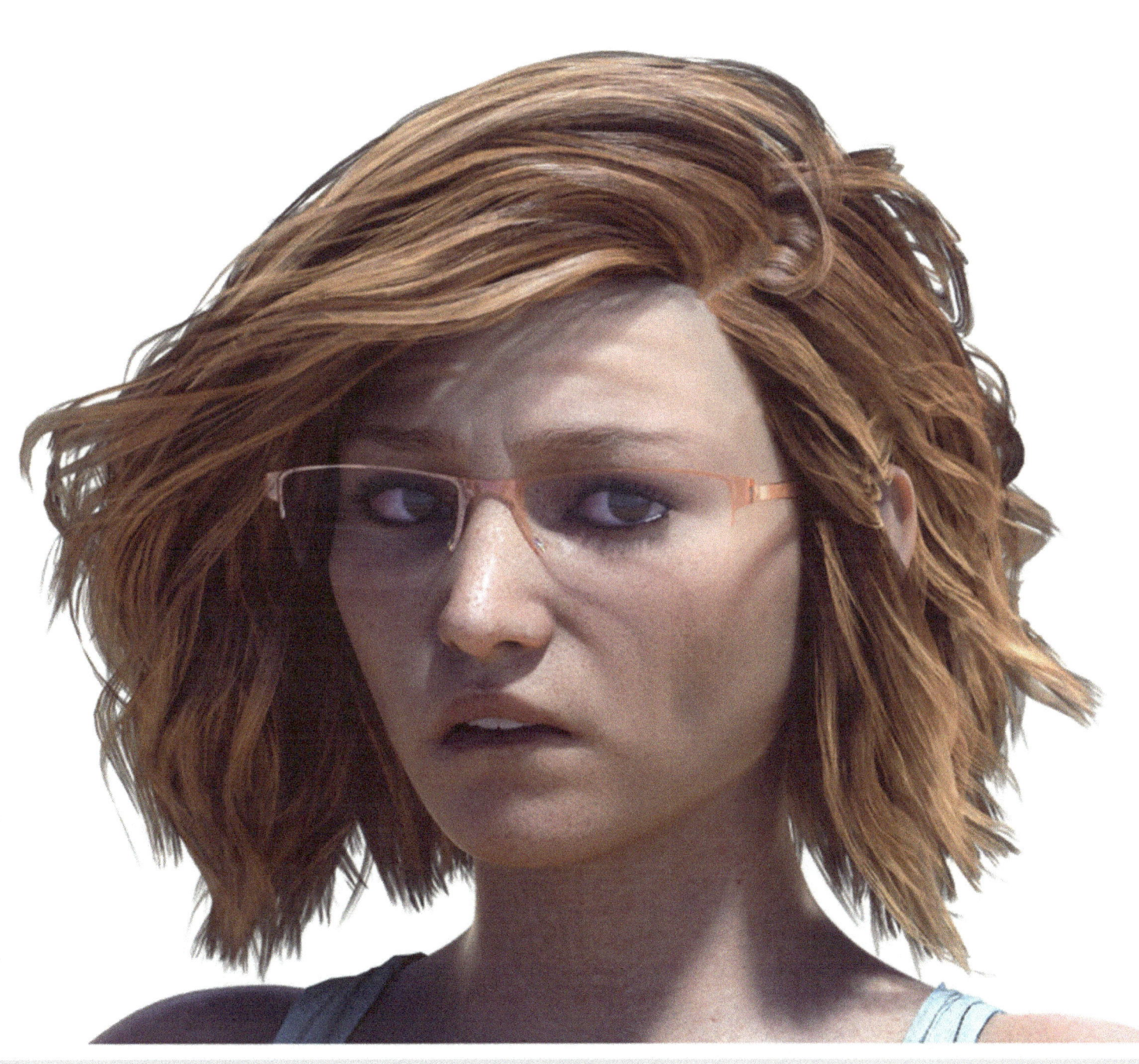

You are all children of the light and of the day; we don't belong to darkness and night.
1 THESSALONIANS 5:5

While you are experiencing hair loss, remember to love on yourself. Do not be hard on yourself. Many people are going through something similar in life or perhaps worse. How can you make yourself feel better about your situation? Share a happy thought.

_____

_____

_____

Cut out the negative noise about what others may feel or think about your hair loss or your new experiences. Do not let others dictate your feelings about wearing wigs, toppers, ponytails, extensions, hats, scarves, going natural, etc. You may be surprised at how many people share your same experiences.

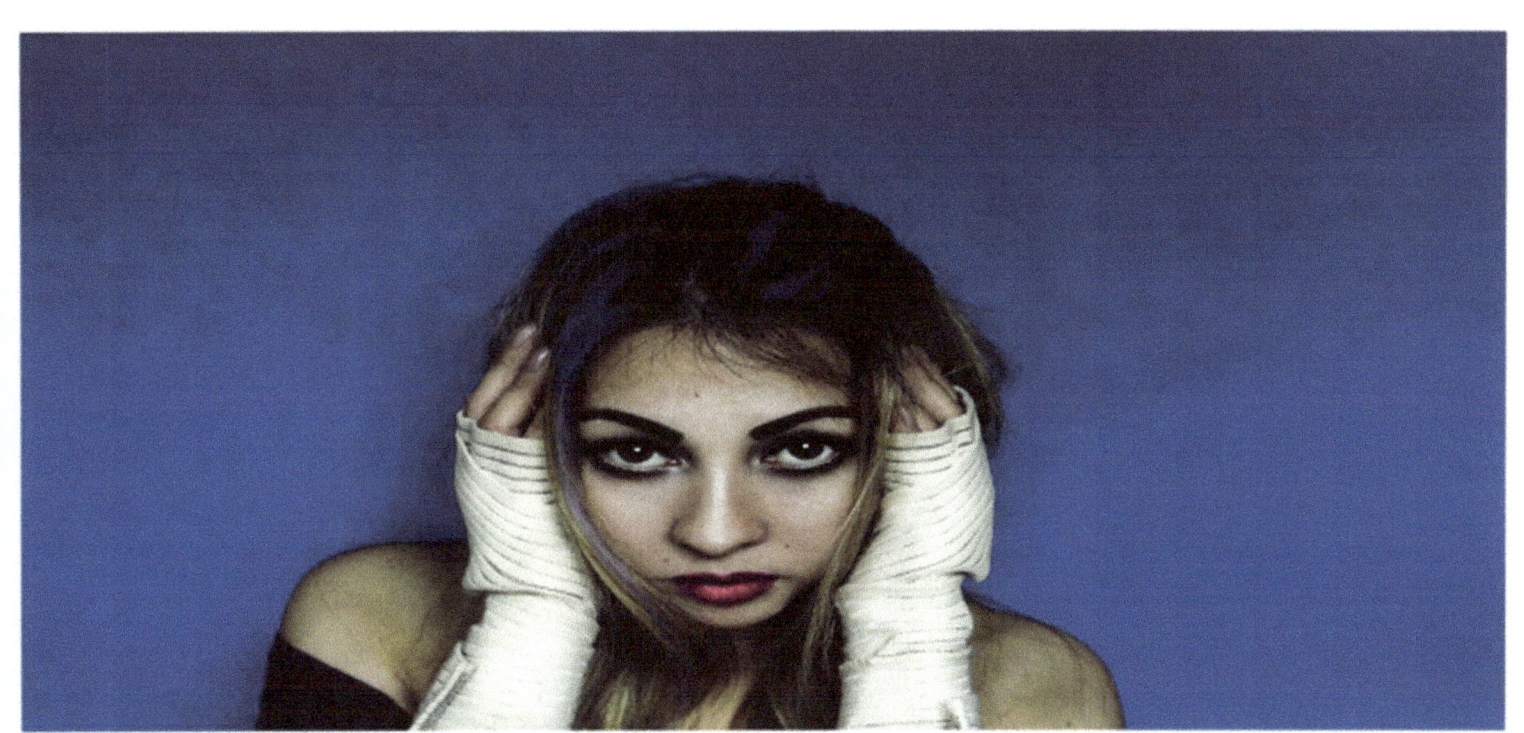

See how very much our Father loves us, for he calls his children, and that is what we are!
1 JOHN 3:1

You are loved! How many people do you know that are experiencing some of what you are going through? Has a relative or friend lost their hair? How did they handle their experience? Can you learn anything from their experiences and apply it to your self-help?

_____

_____

Weeping may last through the night, but joy comes with the morning.
PSALM 30: 5

You are enough!

_____

_____

_____

_____

_____

_____

If you love hair, go get some from somewhere and embrace the experience. Make it fun and fulfilling! Name each hairstyle, wig, or topper.

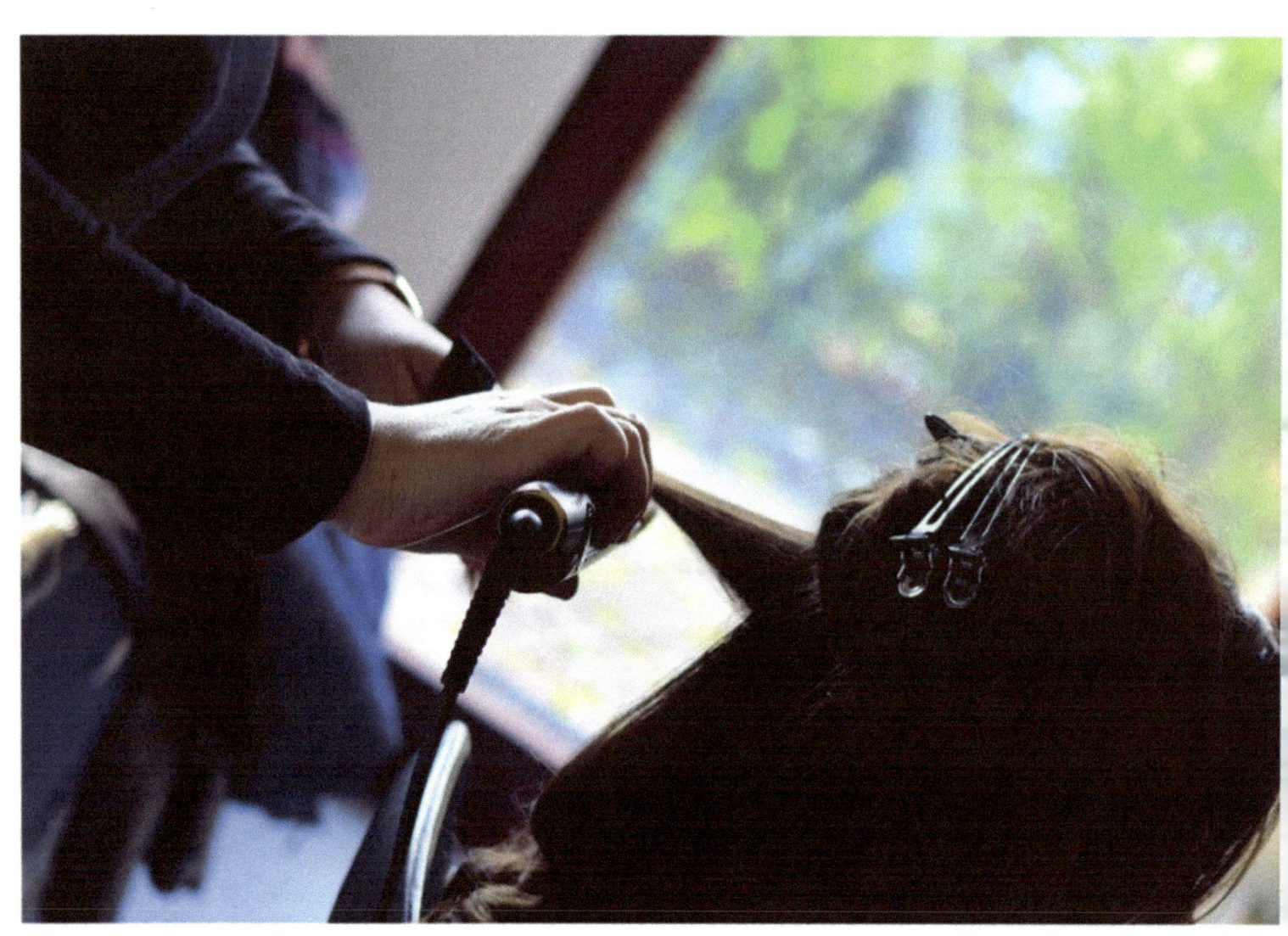

Story time...
Some of us use our hair as a way to experess outwardly what we may be feeling inwardly. A young lady came into my wig store and shared that she had gone through a breakup with a significant other, and as a result of that, she had shaved her head. I thought, "Why?" I then asked her if cutting her hair felt freeing? She agreed that cutting her hair freed her from the old and tramatic experience of the breakup. She came into the wig store to restore her hair with a new wig. She needed "Mo-Nu Hair!"

"I Know the plans I have for you," says the Lord. "They are plans for good and not for disaster, to give you a future and a hope."
JEREMIAH 29: 11

Do you use your hair as a means of expression? How have you done so? How did it make you feel?

_____

_____

_____

_____

_____

_____

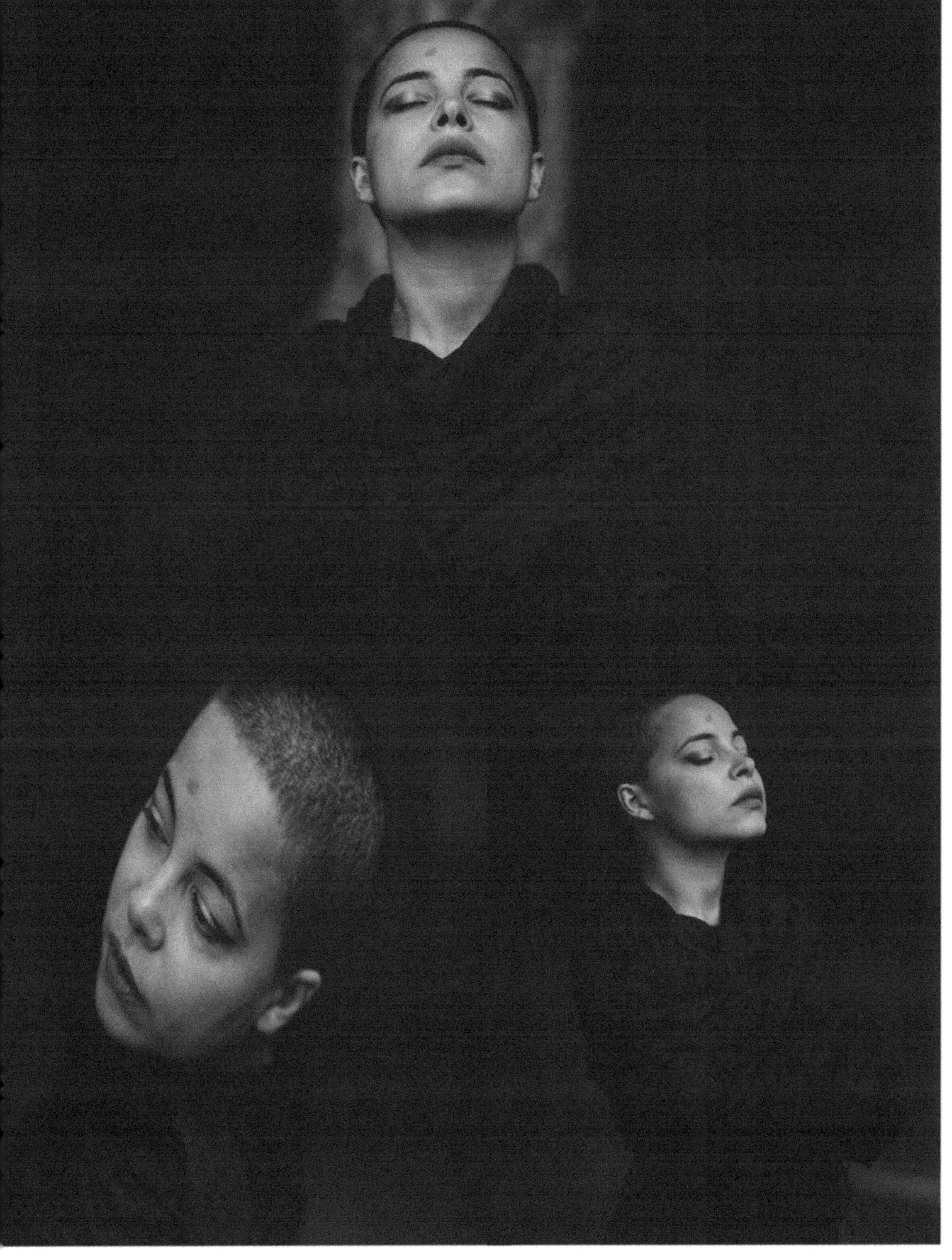

God is love, and all who live in love
live in God, and God lives in them.
1 JOHN 4:16

_____

_____

_____

_____

_____

_____

_____

_____

_____

_____

Short hair, long hair, colored hair, shaved hair, and no hair- It is not just hair! Oftentimes, hair speaks to us. But no matter what your hair may be saying to you at the moment, it is simply apart of who you are, and not who you are as a whole person.

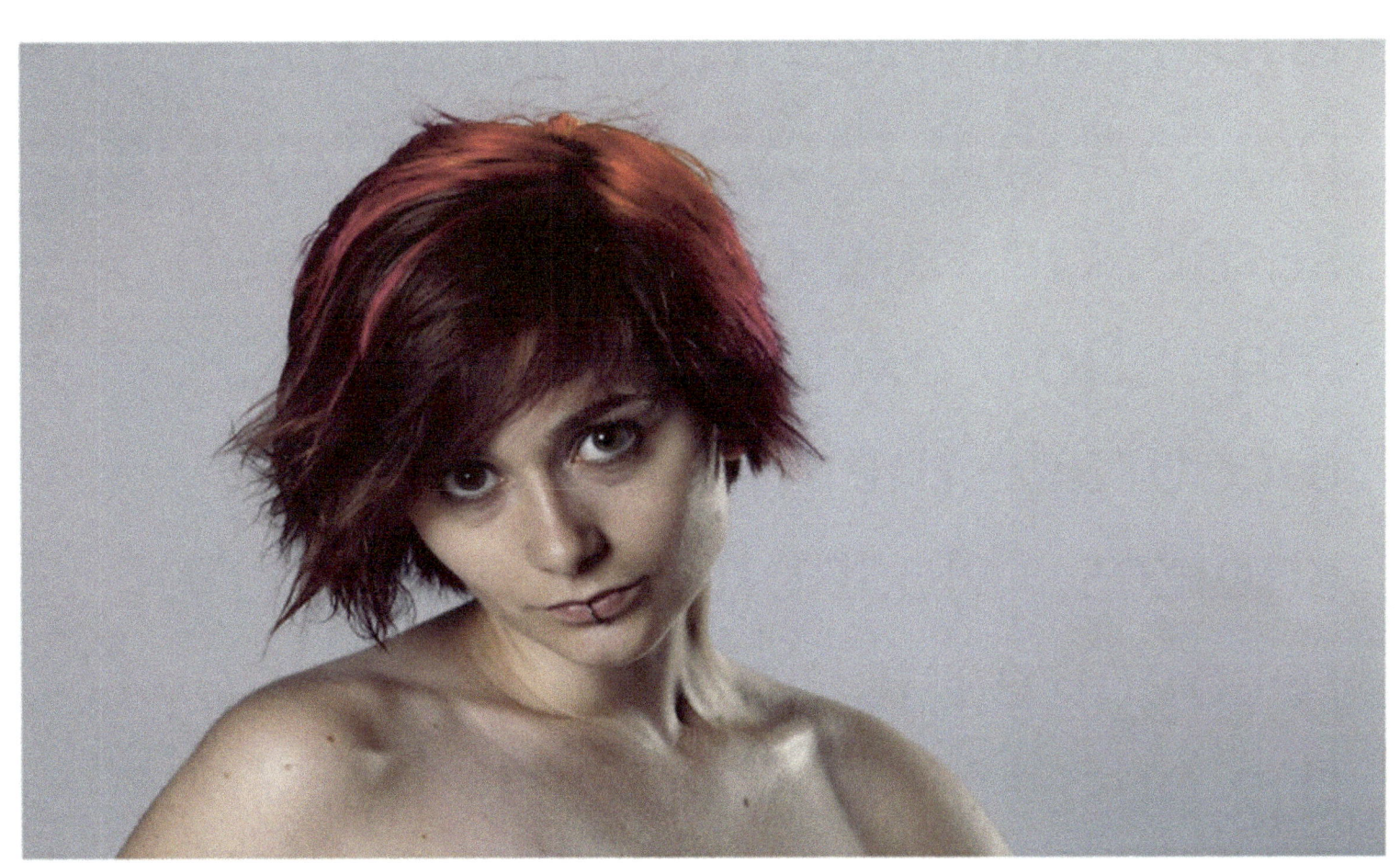

DAUGHTERS (Teens)

Daughters can be very supportive of their loved ones that are experiencing hair loss. However, in my experience, there tend to be two different types of reactions from daughters. Teen daughters can be critical of their loved ones' choices in wigs. They want the person that they know to stay the same. On rare occasions, a teen may show excitement and incourage their loved ones wig choices. Most often teens do not recognize the devastation felt by the person experiencing hair loss.

DAUGHTERS (Adults)

Adult daughters can be critical of their loved ones' choices to wear wigs. Some adult daughters feel that hair loss is normal and that embracing the loss is best. Many times, I have heard daughters say in demanding tones, "You do not need a wig!" or Why do you want a wig?" On the other hand, there are daughters who are empathetic towards their loved ones' choice to wear wigs. They are motivational caring, with genuine concerns about their loved ones feelings regarding hair loss.

Husbands...

Husbands are supportive. They affirm their wives. They also know what looks good on their wives. It is apparent that many husbands seek happiness for their wives as their wives experience hair loss. I have witnessed unconditional love in many couples.

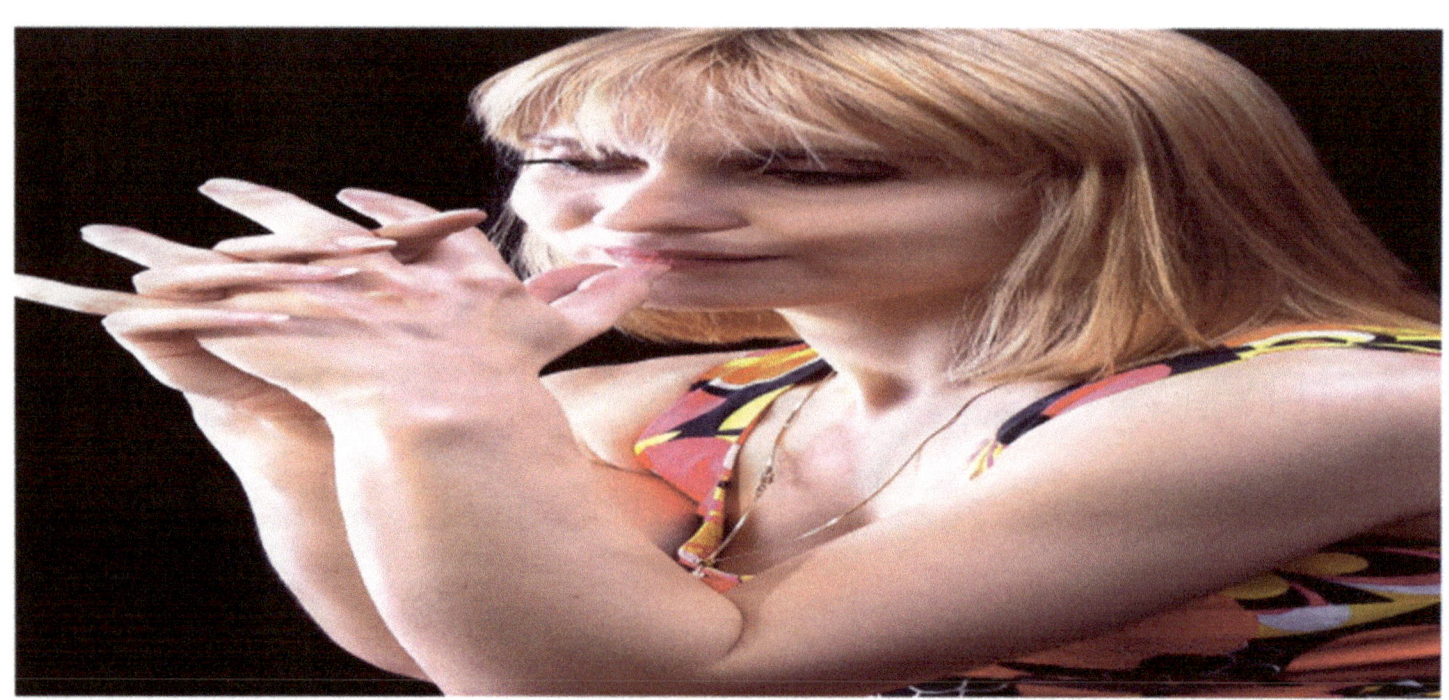

Support system

What type of support system do you have? Make sure that you surround yourself with people that are caring, loving and supportive of your hair loss experience.

_____

_____

_____

_____

_____

Mothers

Mothers want to find a solution to the problem. They are vocal about their loved ones' hair loss. Mothers are encouraging, but can also be slightly opinionated when it comes to hair replacement choices. They remember what their daughters' hair used to be like and tend to lean toward finding the same colors and styles that they are used to seeing on their loved ones.

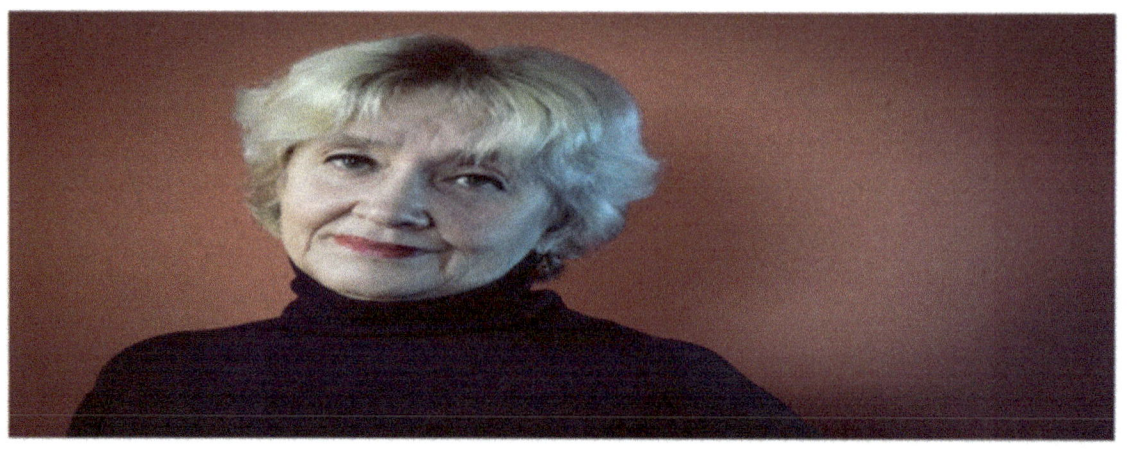

"Will my hair ever be the same as it was before I started experiencing hair loss?" "I just want my hair back!" "I had such beautiful hair."
"I am looking for something that looks like my hair." These are some comments that I hear daily from my wig-wearing community. This is when I redirect the conversation in a more realistic but positive direction. I say, "We are embracing newness." Oftentimes, family members agree with me. Fathers have been most supportive of their daughters.

FATHERS

Story Time...

Moe came to check out wigs before her hair would be cut off. She was preparing to get a wig before her cancer treatments started. She came in with her boyfriend and her father. I was impressed with how Moe's father was so invested in her choices of wigs. He selected wigs that were very becoming on Moe. As for Moe's boyfriend, he really did not have too much to say about the wig choices. He was supportive of the decisions made by Moe and her father.

Insensitivity

Sometimes those who are the closest to us are our worse critics. We are critical enough about ourselves. It is difficult to swallow criticism from people that are considered confidants. I was told that a husband told his wife, whose hair was thinning, "You look like a cancer patient." This was hurtful and disrepectful on so many levels. The heartless comment suggested that the man's wife had a choice in her hair loss situation. Also, his comment was not empathetic towards the cancer community.

Words can be used to uplift or discourage spirits. Let us remember the beauty in kindness to others and ourselves.

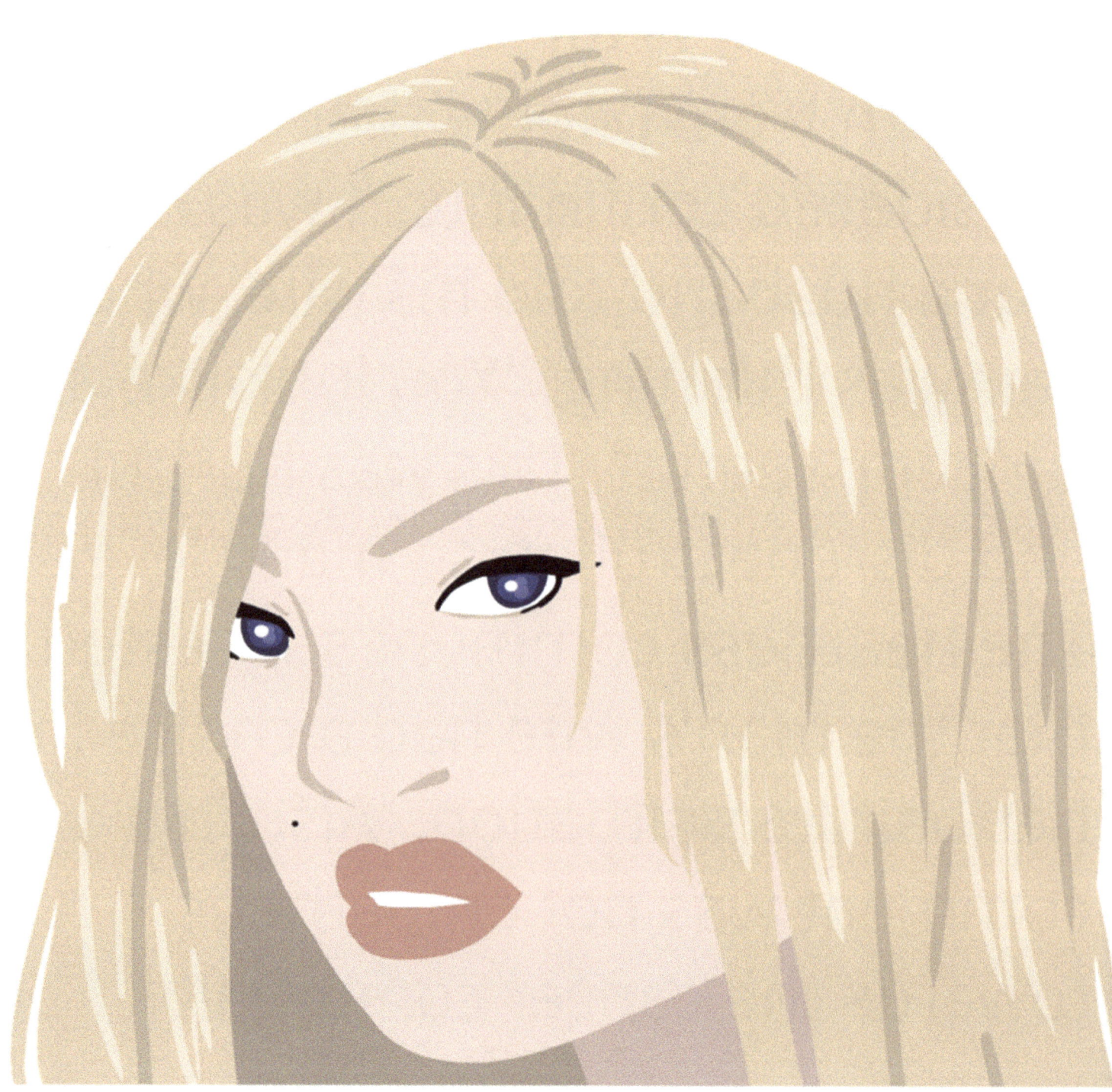

Hair Follicle...

What is the hair follicle and how does it aid in hair growth?

The follicle is an opening in the skin through which the hair grows. Each hair follicle anchors a hair of the skin. The hair bulb, which is at the end of each strand of hair, forms the base of the hair follicle. The hair bulb is made up of living cells that divide and grow, building the hair shaft. Blood vessels supply nourishment and hormones to the bulb. The hormones modify the hair's growth and structure at different times of life.

That white tip at the end of the hair shaft is called the bulb. This bulb is made up of a keratin protein. It forms the hair at the bottom of the follicle and roots the hair to the scalp. The 4.16 mm follicle and bulb allows the hair to feed from the supplied nourishment and hormones until the hair falls out.

Scalp messages, hair serums and cleansers can promote the follicles to react through stimulation and nourishment.

There are so many products that are promoted in order to address the needs of people with hair loss. It can be frustrating to put hope in expensive miracle treatments. Every day, I am asked about what products can be used in order to reverse hair loss. I always asked the person about their person health concerns. Hair loss is often related to known and unknown health issues, medications or stress. It is true that certain topical creams and medication can help, but I would advise getting a doctors opinion on hair loss concerns.

Experiencing the loss of hair can be a traumatic ordeal. However, you are more than your hair. You have value that is far beyond your hair. Never forget your worth. Learn all that you can about hair and teach someone else. Someone can benefit from your experience.

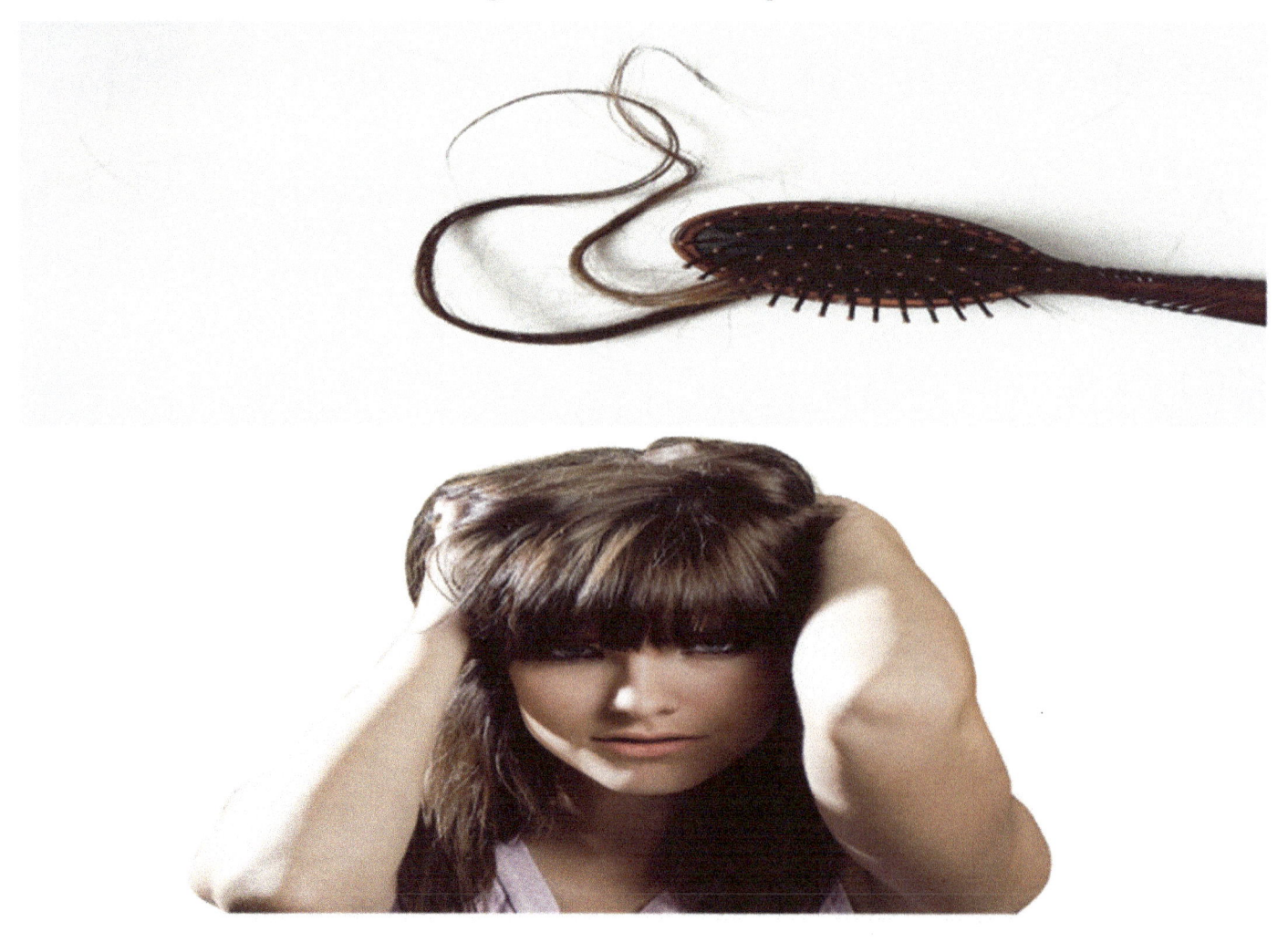

Covid 19
Story Time...
Many women have shared with me how their hair has been affected by Covid-19.
They have testified to their hair feeling different. Some said that their hair thinned or fell out in clumps. A teen girl told me that her hair loss had occurred as a result of having Covid-19, mononucleosis, and streptococcus all at once. She had no hair at all on the crown of her head. She wore a baseball cap in order to cover her baldness.

The thing that I appreciated about this young teen was that she was not discouraged about her hair loss. She was very positive and full of life. I was surprised by her enthusiasm. She did not like being bald, but she did not let her hair loss put her into a depression or make her withdrawn. She tried on several wigs, but did not find one that she liked. She was content to keep wearing her hat until she found the right look for her. I was very proud of this young lady. She did not allow her circumstances to dictate her mood in a negative way.

Gastric Bypass, Metabolic or Bariatric Surgery...

It is common for people to experience hair loss after a few months of having a weight-loss surgery. Not getting enough dietary nutrients including protein, will cause hair loss. Losing weight rapidly stresses the body. Nutrient deficiencies damage the root of the hair. When the hair tries to grow, it breaks while trying to get through the scalp. The body needs 60 to 80 grams of protein daily, as well as zinc, potassium, vitamin B6, or phosphorus and biotin. Consult with your doctor.

It is believed that hair loss due to weight-loss surgeries, is not permanent. The hair will grow back. To minimize the loss, consuming the necessary proteins, vitamins, and minerals can help. Be sure to eat a variety of healthy foods always.

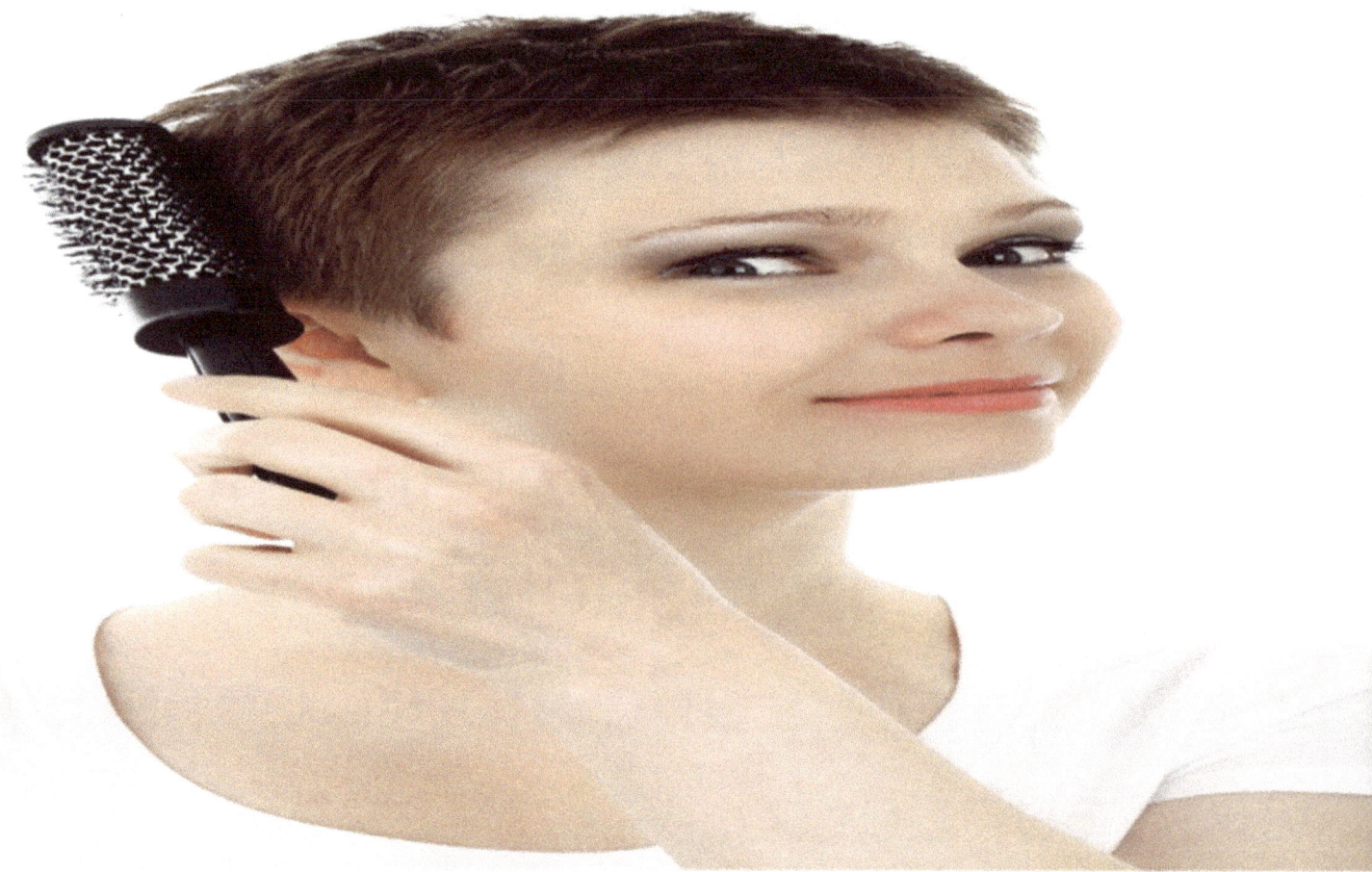

Hair loss can result from both type 1 and type 2 diabetes. However, getting your diabetes under control can help to prevent hair loss. Health is critical to healthy scalp and hair.

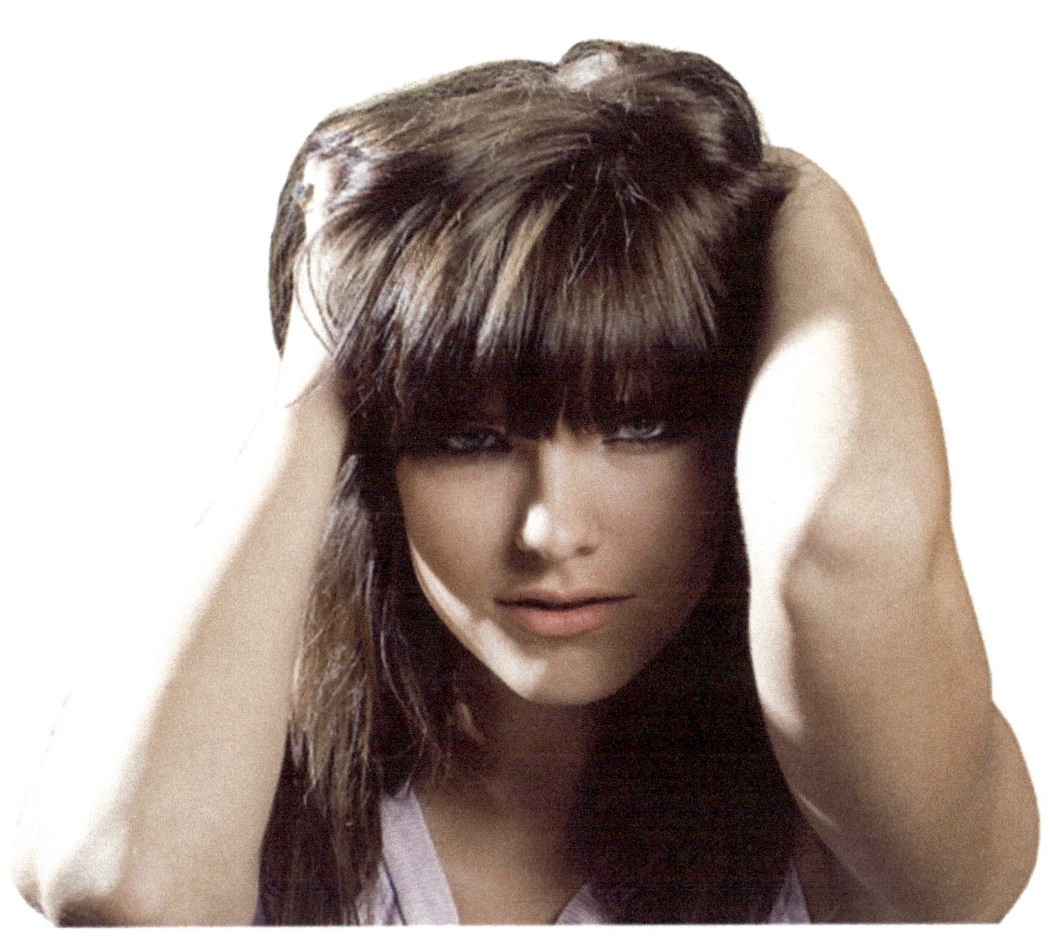

This book aims to encourage you to overcome the fears, depressions, and anxieties that you may be feeling as a result of losing your hair. Understanding that you are not alone is the point of this journey. There are many others, both women and men, that experience hair loss at different times of their lives. Although it is not a pleasant experience, it is not something that should keep you from the joy of life. Be free in your spirit and overcome your new change by embracing the hair loss as a new experience that you may learn, teach, and grow from.

Do Nots...

>Do not give up on yourself because of the hair loss.

>Do not let hair loss defeat you.

>Do not allow the hair loss to consume your thoughts.

>Do not let the hair loss make you feel less than who you have always been.

The do nots can continue, but I think that the point has been made. Losing hair is hard enough; do not allow the hair loss to keep you hiding physically or mentally. Find ways to overcome the hair loss. Be open to new ways of beautifying yourself.

Dishing It Out!

It is easy for others to give advice when they themselves have no experience with the subject matter. Advice without experience can be annoying. I do not want to be preachy or annoying. I have certainly experienced my own hair loss. My hair loss had been chronic for many years. I never knew why. I worried about the loss continously. My hair would lightly shed. I used relaxers and assumed that relaxing my hair was the culprit. However, after stopping the use of relaxers, I continued to have minimal hair loss.

As a young adult, I did not consider how important a factored my overall health was tob my hair loss. I was always on some type of fad diet. I did not take vitamins, or supplements, and did not drink enough water on a regular basis. Looking back on my daily nutritional care, I think it is a wonder that I had any hair at all. My hair grew, but was very fragile.

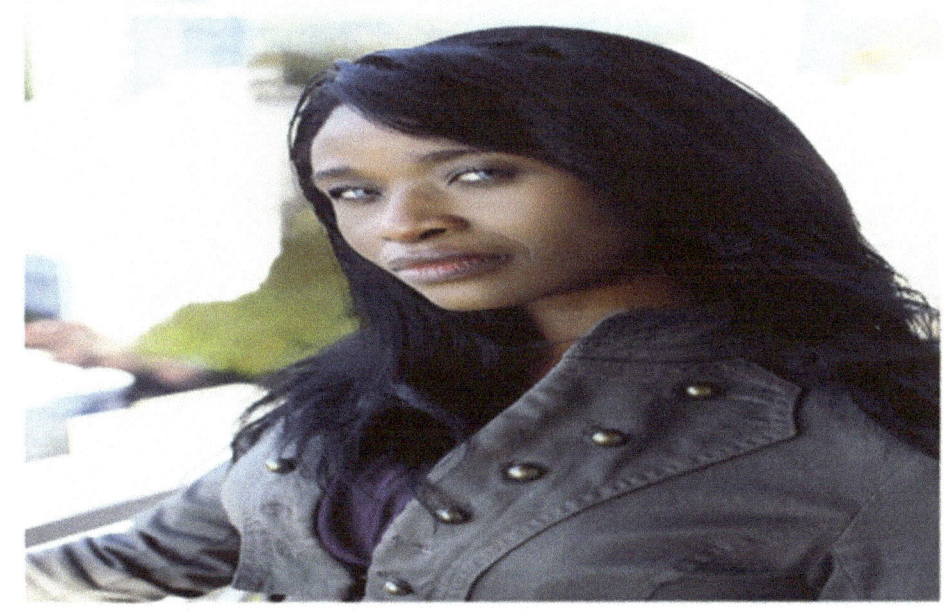

I was affraid to handle my hair. I felt stressed just thinking about having to touch it. I knew that stressing about my hair loss was not helping at the matter, though, so I decided to let the shedding take place without my worrying about it. I was grateful for the hair that held in my scalp. However, I do admit that it was very difficult not to think about the lost hairs. Fortunately, I was always able to braid my hair and not worry about losing hair while it was in a protective style.

After turning fifty, the edges of my hair started thinning. Wearing glasses that pulled on the sides of my hair did not help. I thought, "Wow, this hair issue never ends." Losing hair can make you feel miserable, self-conscious and distressed. I wanted to give up. But give up on what? Myself? My life? What does it mean to give up?" Well for me it acutually meant to take a stand of not letting it worry me anymore. There is nothing that can be done about getting older and losing hair. I decided to embrace the new me. If that meant cutting my hair off and starting fresh, or wearing wigs, I was for it. No more concerning myself with an issue that I had not control over. I decided to have fun with hair that comes packaged. I decided I would like to have great styling hair. Hair that I could do anything with, take all of the abuse that I could put it through and still grow. Wouldn't that be wonderful? However, that is not realistic. Therefore, I will make due and be content with what I have, fragile and temperamental hair. I love you hair.

Hair Hurt Harms Heart...

"4H" stands for Hair Hurt Harms Heart. Many people feel brokenhearted when their hair is not at its best. Feeling alone, some people isolate while going through hair-hurting experiences. One of my clients wore a sweat shirt stating "Home Body." She did not feel normal and stays home as ofter as possible. When she got her new wig, she was elated. At one point during the wig install she teared up. There may have been other reasons for her tears, but certainly hair hurt was a reason.

Hair Ministries is what my wig/salon shop should be called. Hurts about hair tramas get shared. Discovering potential solutions, hair goals, and recoveries is at the heart of the matter.

I would like to thank all of my clients and my wig wearing community for sharing their stories. Talking and journaling about experiences can be triggering. It is also theraputic and can assist in the healing process. I would also like to send love and blessings to all of you. Thrive!

Hair Loss Info and Cancer Centers

Cancer Hot Line...800-227-2345

African American Cancer Patients...888-793-9355

Grants for Cancer...888-261-4837

Cancer Care for Children...800-813-4673

WebMD.com/hair-loss

ClevelandClinic.org...216-444-4004

Thank you for your interest in learning more about hair and the psychology of hair through my experiences and the shared experiences of others. If there is anything that I can help you with, please reach out to me at MO-NU HAIR CITY. I have been called the "Wig Doctor."; I love that! It shows me that people value my insight about their hair needs.
NorthTown Mall,
4750 N. Division St. #1234
Spokane WA. 99207

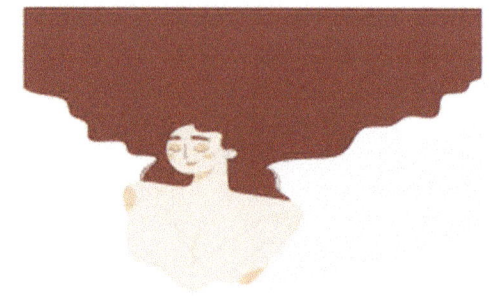

Ingram Content Group UK Ltd.
Milton Keynes UK
UKHW051114260523
422386UK00008B/23